MW00801014

IT WASN'T SUPPOSED TO BE LIKE THIS

A Postpartum Depression Survival Guide With Over 100 Ideas to Manage Loneliness, Sadness and Guilt So You Can Begin to Enjoy Motherhood

LAURIE VARGA

brain
sugar
MEDIA

Copyright © 2021 by Laurie Varga

All rights reserved. This book or any portion thereof may not be reproduced or used in any manner whatsoever without the express written permission of the publisher except for the use of brief quotations in a book review.

Although the author and publisher have made every effort to ensure that the information in this book was correct at production time, the author and publisher do not assume and hereby disclaim any liability to any party for any loss, damage, or disruption caused by errors or omissions, whether such errors or omissions result from negligence, accident, or any other cause.

This book is not intended as a substitute for professional medical advice. Please consult a physician in matters relating to your physical and mental health, particularly with respect to any symptoms that may require diagnosis or medical attention. If you believe you are at risk of hurting yourself, your child, or anyone else, please consult a medical professional or helpline immediately.

ISBN 978-0-9948159-3-4

www.ppdbook.com

Cover images: iStock.com | Design: Laurie Varga

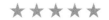

Reviews

"I wish I had a guide like this to walk me through the fog. I saw myself reflected in the pages, reminding me how hard this was, not only for me but for my partner and family. The humor sprinkled throughout added a necessary lightness."

– Mother of two, San Diego, CA

"This book should be given to every first-time mom."

– Mother of one, Mississauga, ON

"Written with such raw honesty it feels like a breath of fresh air during a time of great pain, desperation and struggle. Laurie has an ability to speak openly and find words for things that feel impossible to think, let alone to say out loud."

– Mother of two, Waterloo, ON

"This book gave me the permission to look at my experience and recall that there were tears (and some joy) for parenting a newborn child had many emotions and colors. The tools and aids that she has listed are helpful and authentic."

– Mother of two, New York City, NY

""If you know someone experiencing PPD, read this as a window into how they might be feeling and how you might be able to help."

– A loving aunt, Toronto, ON

To all the honest women I've met
And the ones I haven't yet
had the pleasure of meeting

CONTENTS

36. Breathe

37. Stop listening to self-help gurus

38. Clean

39. Tackle one small project that has been bugging you for ages

40. Brighten up your life

41. Spend time in nature

42. Take a course

43. Be spontaneous

44. Send kind notes to people you've neglected

45. Hug someone

46. Talk to strangers

47. Give something

48. Receive a foot massage

49. Blow up your stress

50. Stretch

51. Say goodbye

52. Early to bed

53. Take things one day minute at a time

54. Change your hair

55. Wear your best clothes

56. Wear your PJs

57. Pick an interesting historical figure and read their biography

58. Make someone else look good

59. Do nothing

60. Play with kid's toys

61. Invite a friend over for a game

62. Tell someone how much they mean to you

63. Read the Velveteen Rabbit

64. Say no

65. Say yes

66. Let me think about it

67. Try new food

68. Take a looong shower

69. Get a white board for the bathroom

70. Call a random person from your address book

71. As soon as you think of a person—call them

72. Send a postcard or a letter

73. Find a local waterfall

74. Go to a performance for a band you've never heard of

75. Have sex

76. Eat something you love

77. Write a song

78. Let go of success

79. Ask unusual questions

80. Fall in love

81. Want what you already have

82. See the gift in your struggle

83. Give some more

84. Memorize something

85. Do something weird

86. Everything is better by candlelight

87. Take extra good care of yourself

88. Sleep in

89. Go slow

90. Stop explaining

91. Collage

92. Compare leads to despair

93. Change your mind

94. Don't take advice

95. Know your values

96. Share something deep

97. Smile

98. Solve a puzzle

99. Don't answer

100. Play the love game

101. Plant seeds

102. Invest in earplugs

103. Receive

104. Little luxuries

105. Hitting the wall

106. Befriend other species

107. Do it your way

108. Just exist

The end

Free reader bonus

Before you go

Read this first

When we find ourselves hanging by a thin thread, scraping our way through rough times, it's easy to forget the small but essential things that keep us sane.

Like breathing.

Despite the fact that I have spent many years studying various breathing techniques, I still forget how to breathe when I'm stressed. I figure most of us could use a few reminders and maybe some new ideas for coping with what seems to be nearly impossible at times.

Initially, I created this list as a personal guide to help me get through the most harrowing event I've ever endured, the birth of my son. At times I couldn't remember things like my own anniversary, let alone perform necessary care procedures like brushing my teeth. So, this list was born.

The content on these pages is not groundbreaking, but it may help if you're willing to experiment. You might even find some relief in having read bits and pieces of it and in knowing that there are others out there who understand the hell you're trudging through.

Most of the ideas here do not require significant investments of capital or time. Many can even be managed by someone as wigged out, exhausted, and weepy as a new parent.

You can be creative in how you use this book. Here are a few suggestions:

- Try out one item each day for 100+ days

- Flip through the book and pick out a handful of ideas that appeal to you and add them to your daily life for a few days or a few weeks

- Close your eyes, open the book to any page, and point to something

- Or any other way you want to use this book that makes you feel good.

Laurie

March 2021

You are not alone

If you have ever felt isolated
from your friends, other mothers, loved ones, or your child

You are not alone

If you have ever been afraid
you might harm yourself or your child

You are not alone

If you have ever wanted to die
that the pain might finally subside

You are not alone

If you have worried
you're the worst parent in the world

You are not alone

If you have felt unworthy
to have this responsibility, this gift of life

You are not alone

If you have ever felt guilty
that you're not doing enough, that you aren't enough

You are not alone

If you have wanted to run
If you have wanted to disappear

You are not alone

If you have ever believed
your child would be better off without you

You are not alone

If you fear
you may have made a terrible mistake

You are not alone

And you are welcome in the fold of these pages.
These words are for you, because many of us know even if
we don't say it aloud:

We are with you.

Why I wrote this

It could have been about 2 am. My son may have been a year old or maybe younger. Or was he older? I can't recall. It's hard to remember much of anything when you've gone months or more without a solid sleep.

Now I understand why sleep deprivation is used as a torture technique; it destroys people.

Sometimes it inspires them to write books like this one. During the first few years postpartum, my mind resembled the simple bowls of mush I fed my kid. There wasn't much I could do with my lack of time, sleep, and sanity except make a simple list. I needed a mental boot camp. So, I decided to write down as many ways to cope with postpartum depression as I could think of.

I figured it might take me a month to come up with 100 ways. It took a few days, and then I thought of a few more.

It wasn't that I had practiced all of these ideas, and it wasn't that I intended to make them part of my life, but instead, it was a way to make a feeble return to the world of the non-zombies. A way to (hopefully) pull me back from the edge of the cliff that I found myself approaching daily. The cliff was a dangerous place to stand. A place you ventured toward only when you didn't want to live anymore—a place where there existed the possibility of freedom from the chains of motherhood.

That freedom came with the responsibility of abandoning everyone else in my life, especially my son. At times, this intense fear was the thin thread that kept me a few steps away from the fatal edge. I reached out to various places for help, but there was little I could rely on. I was armed with prescription drugs and my willpower, nothing more. With these simple tools, I started to write.

If you're wondering where I found the time, let's just say that's one of the only benefits to insomnia.

Once I had my list, the next logical step was to elaborate on them to understand them better. As I filled out the paragraphs, it occurred that these ramblings might help others with depression. In the beginning, I kept the ideas and title generic because I was afraid to be too forward about the topic of depression, suicide—and especially—postpartum depression.

It took years to come to terms with what this book was about, and a few more months to write an honest preface. Because if there's one illness you can't be frank about, it's PPD. When my son was about a month old, I called a postpartum crisis line. I remember the woman on the phone asking me what I liked about being a mother. I enjoyed nothing about it at the time, but I made something up out of fear they'd commit me or take my son away.

It's strange how all I thought I wanted was not to be a parent anymore, but I couldn't take it when presented with the option.

I'm an expert in self-inflicted misery.

I hope you enjoy reading this and that you feel better soon.

Free reader bonus

As a thank you for perusing this book, I've created free bonus material, including a personal video.

Please visit **https://www.ppdbook.com/reader-bonus** to access your goodies.

Get Some Sleep

[Note: This idea is rather dull, and I apologize for that. BUT it is likely the most essential idea in this book and one of the best tools I know of for restoring mental balance.]

Although the sleep issue is evident for many parents, it helps to be reminded that sleep deprivation is used in war as a form of torture. You are not delusional if a sleepless child is holding you hostage.

You are not weird for choosing a nap over lunch with Hugh Jackman (as you crawl to your bed in your plaid PJs).

I'm not going to tell you that the good news is some kids grow out of it, because some of them don't. By the time my son was seven years old, it still took hours to get him to sleep, and he woke up almost every night.

I want to let you know that your sleep is more than just important; it's critical. Although we still don't know much about the purpose of sleep, the latest research suggests it's a mechanism for restoring the brain. Sleep is not so much a physical activity (or lack thereof) but a mental one. When we fail to get enough sleep, particularly over a period of time, it is likely to contribute to, or aggravate, mental illnesses like depression and anxiety.[1]

As parents, we often don't get to choose when we sleep and for how long. This lack of control can be further aggravated by insomnia, creating a downward spiral of sleeplessness and despair.

---

1   Jakke Tamminen, "4 Ways Not Getting Enough Sleep Affects Your Brain." The Independent, Independent Digital News and Media, October 17, 2016. Accessed March 20, 2020 at www.independent.co.uk/life-style/health-and-families/how-a-lack-of-sleep-affects-you-brain-from-your-personality-to-how-you-learn-a7366216.html.

I've been there—many times—and not all the tricks in my toolbox work consistently. I tend to lean toward natural remedies as much as possible. When they fail, the demons in my mind amplify like a nasty real-life video game. Then I pull the big guns out of my bedside table.

These words are here to remind you of the necessity to take care of yourself. Ignore what other people have to say about your choices. As my dear friend's wise mother said:

"Your opinion is none of my business."

Here are a few tips from a fellow insomniac who has tried almost everything:[2]

- Develop a slow, soothing bedtime routine.

- Go to bed at the same time your child does. (This happens by accident quite frequently, I find).

- Turn off your computer & phone at least 1 hour before bedtime. You don't need to check the news, your social feeds, or your e-mail before you check out.

- Take calcium/magnesium right before you go to bed. I discovered this by accident, and it works quite well, although I've found I need to take my vitamins for a few consecutive nights for it to kick in.

- Take melatonin about 45-60 minutes before you go to bed. Melatonin is a naturally occurring hormone in animals (including us). It helps regulate sleep patterns, and I've found it very helpful for knocking me out when I'm struggling to ease into sleep. Begin with the smallest dose possible, usually 0.5-1mg. If it's ineffective for a couple of nights, add another milligram. Too

---

2 Although Tim Ferriss, author of The 4-Hour Workweek, swears by taking an ice-cold bath before bed it sounds absolutely dreadful, so I've skipped that one. Also, what does he know? He doesn't have kids.

much melatonin can leave you feeling sluggish during the day, so the less you take, the better you'll feel in the morning. I take about 0.5mg and have found that small amount to do the trick.[3]

- Snuggle under warm covers in a cool room.

- Try a head-to-toe relaxation exercise before bed.

- If you're on medication, it might be affecting your sleep. I experienced this and switched the timing of one of my meds. Talk to your doctor about making adjustments if you think your medication might be an issue.

- A soothing cup of caffeine-free sleepy tea is often helpful.

- Avoid alcohol before bed. Although it may make you sleepy, it disrupts sleep patterns, and many people tend not to sleep well under the influence.

- Do what's necessary for you to get a night of good sleep, even if that means sleeping with your child. Or sleeping without them if that works. Your mental health is essential; do not put other people's ideas about what is best for you ahead of your own when it comes to sleep.

- Block out noise with simple foam earplugs (I use them most nights), a white noise machine, fan, or other devices. Don't worry about not hearing your kid; they don't work that well.

- Ask someone else to keep an eye on your little one(s) while you rest. The worst thing they can say is "no."

- Download a sleep hypnosis app for your phone or stream one online.

---

3   Note that it's not advisable to take melatonin for more than a few weeks as it may reduce your body's own production of this essential hormone. See: "Melatonin for Sleep: Does It Work?" Johns Hopkins Medicine. Accessed February 9, 2021 at https://www.hopkinsmedicine.org/health/wellness-and-prevention/melatonin-for-sleep-does-it-work.

- Put your child in a safe place (cribs are handy for this) and put in earphones while listening to gentle music or waves. Even if your babe is pitching a fit, it's okay. A physician I know, a mother of two young kids herself, reassured me:

"No baby ever died from crying."

Be honest

I've always wanted to have the courage to be honest. I wanted to be bold with people—to have the cojones to say what everyone else is thinking like a straight-talking Scottish nana.

Studies conducted by psychologist Robert S. Feldman reveal the average person lies about two or three times per 10 minutes of conversation.[4] That's a lot of fibbing. You might be trying to convince yourself this stat doesn't apply to you, but that could very well be lie number 132 today. We lie about many little things like telling someone how much we love the itchy scarf they made us for Christmas or pretending we're okay when we're falling apart. Little white lies erode our sense of self.

An excellent place to start with this honesty business is by examining the lies we tell ourselves.

There is no need to be cruel or brutal in order to be honest with ourselves and others, but it isn't easy at first. It requires acceptance of our vulnerability and the creation of a new habit at the same time. I suggest, for just one day, to be honest whenever you think of it. Notice the way an untruth feels in your body. Do you feel it in your chest, your

---

4   Robert S. Feldman, University of Massachusetts Amherst, "UMass Amherst Researcher Finds Most People Lie in Everyday Conversation", June 10, 2002. Accessed March 9, 2021 at https://www.umass.edu/newsoffice/article/umass-amherst-researcher-finds-most-people-lie-everyday-conversation

stomach, or your jaw? Take a breath, notice the raw emotions at the core of the issue (if you have the time and space), then speak to those real sensations instead of reverting to the automatic impulse to cover up the truth.

If I were to be upfront right now, I'm worried this idea is bland and uninspiring. I'm afraid to save it. I'm just going to squeeze my eyes shut and do it.

Purge

Permit yourself to discard things that don't make you feel good. If there's guilt, resentment, anger, or any lousy feeling associated with some tangible item in your life, toss it.

You don't need to do a full house scan and discard 20 big black bags. Just a shopping bag is a good start. Throw out things you find while digging around in the back of the pantry, or when you open your closet to reveal that shirt you never wear for a million reasons.

The stuff you don't love is clogging up your head and your heart, dragging you down like a rusty anchor. If you want newer, better things to come into your life, you have to make space for them.

I have a divorced friend who wanted to meet the right guy and get married again but struggled to find appropriate husband material. It occurred to her that the old wedding dress from her first marriage was still taking up space in her closet and her life. If there's already one dress in there, it's pretty tough to squeeze in a second, so she donated the mass expanse of white silk to make room for a new one.

Of course, I wouldn't be sharing this story if it didn't work, and today, she is happily married with two kids.

Old, unused stuff takes up not only physical but emotional and psychological space as well. There are a thousand or more purging methods espoused by people who get paid to organize other people's messes, but the short of it is this: If you haven't used it, needed it, or missed it for six months, it's junk. Get rid of it now. Don't dwell, just toss and move on.

At one point, I went through an aggressive purge over a few months (that's how long it takes when you have a toddler at home all day), and the lightness I felt might have caused me to float away on a windy day. It's all good, though—I'd rather be a kite than a lead weight.

Soak your sins away

I know there are people out there who claim they don't like baths, but I think they're crazy. How could someone not enjoy resting their weary body in a warm, soothing vessel of water? That's like hating puppies.

Fill the tub, add some Epsom salts to relax your muscles, drop in a teaspoon of any random oil to moisturize, light a few candles, and slip in.

Adding a few drops of fragrance is a delightful enhancement too, some lavender or bergamot, perhaps?

If you insist that you're still not a bath person, then have a steaming shower by candlelight. Trust me—it's fantastic. Unless you light the shower curtain on fire.

05

Drink tea

Considering the length of its popularity around the globe, I think it's safe to say there is something special about tea. Even Kermit the Frog dedicated a News Flash to the historical Boston Tea Party. It was a moving bit of journalism.

Whether a quiet cup on the front porch or shared with a group of friends and a deck of cards, tea is a lovely way to sip your worries away. Unless the game is poker and you're losing. Regardless of the kind of tea, each has its own physical and psychological effects. I could go on about the health benefits of antioxidants and caffeine, but I'd rather just wrap my hands around a warm mug of Earl Grey.

A few years ago, during my survivalist phase (hey, we all have some eyebrow-raising hobbies in our personal history), I took a workshop to learn how to build an emergency snow shelter; a key skill one needs when living in Canada. The instructor emphasized the importance of first creating a small fire to keep us warm and motivated. He would then boil some water for tea, sit back, and decide how best to build his shelter. I liked this guy right away.

Taking a step back with a warm beverage in hand struck me as a brilliant idea for rescuing ourselves from any kind of high-stress situation.

In times of duress, our ability to think clearly and perform optimally are diminished. We might be tempted to believe that getting down to work right away is the best strategy, but sometimes clearing our head with a warm cup of tea might just be the best course of action.

I'm going to make myself a cup right now...

Note: I am well aware of how hard it can be to achieve even this simple task within parenthood's confines. When my son was a baby, he was so demanding I could not complete the process of making tea from start to finish on some days. Actually, on many days. That was a dark time.

If you can find someone to bring you tea—god bless them.

06

Avoid the sauce

Some studies swear by the health benefits of red wine, and other health advocates swear off booze altogether. It's interesting to note that multiple studies indicate people on the far end of the spectrum, those who abstain and those who overindulge, have more mental health issues than people who drink in moderation.[5] So why would I suggest you consider maybe not drinking? Because, life is one big laboratory where you get to conduct the experiments. If you typically imbibe in a regular fashion, simply abstain for a few days or a few weeks and see how you feel.

These aren't rules, they're just ideas.

If you think you might have an addiction of any kind, please put your well-being first and reach out to a local counselling service. Talking to someone who is trained to help is a great start.

---

5   "Alcohol and Mental Health." Mental Health Foundation, (Mental Health Foundation of the UK, August 7, 2018.) www.mentalhealth.org.uk/a-to-z/a/alcohol-and-mental-health.

07

Pick up a new hobby

Because you have so much free time as a parent that what you really need is yet another thing to do.

But hear me out, or rather, read a few lines before you discount this one. Your life has been profoundly changed. There are lots of things you used to be able to do that you can't do now, or maybe those things aren't as fun as they used to be like backcountry camping or high-end dining or... sleeping.

It's going to take time to figure out this radical lifestyle, even if it's not your first child. Every new parenting experience is fresh. Unless you're dealing with baby number six, in which case I have to wonder where you're finding the time to read this. Maybe you have some tips to share with the rest of us.

And now that your life is permanently altered, you may want or need to swap out some hobbies for those that are more conducive to where you are now in life. I was quite committed to cycling, kayaking, rappelling, martial arts and yoga before I had my son but with the loss of free time, the loss of my income and a move from a house to an apartment, my regular fitness routine took a huge hit. So, I went out and started doing something I'd not only never done before, it was also something I hated.

Running.

I took up that classic sport that requires nothing but a pair of shoes and some cardio (that I didn't have). I tried running with a jogging stroller, but it was awful—an experience that has been confirmed by other running parents. I ended up running on occasion with the dreaded stroller as well as solo when my husband was home to look after the screamer.

At first it was horrible; I'd curse at myself and everyone else who ever tied a pair of laces. I didn't have enough energy to nod at the other joggers I passed on my pain-inducing journey. But I kept going because I knew I was out of shape and I had hope it would get easier. And it did.

You probably think I'm going to tell you about the marathon I just ran, but you'd be wrong. There's no way in hell I'd ever do that. I can't run more than 5K without sharp pain in my knees, so I usually try to run for about 30-40 minutes, and I take my time to stop and take pictures, another hobby I reacquainted myself with. Turns out there's a fun way to combine both that makes running less of a slog (music also helps).

Whatever this new activity might be for you, experiment, dabble, give it a bit of time and you might find it's something that helps you manage the often-unbearable stress of being a parent. Something that takes the edge off and lets you get to know yourself better.

Have a go at something new or pick up an old hobby you've neglected for other boring things like work and errands. Hobbies have the mojo to deliver enough joy and personal satisfaction to compensate for the time you spend at activities you can't stand like cleaning up vomit, again.

There's no reason you can't get started on your new hobby today. Even if getting started means doing a bit of research. Avoid the trap of losing yourself in endless research (like I often do), the benefit is in the actual doing. Unless your hobby is researching...

There's no right or wrong way to engage in something that lights you up.

08

Walk it off

Movement is good for the body. We weren't designed to spend our days sitting at a desk slumped over a keyboard as I am right now. Like a car, we need to be driven, otherwise we seize up. A simple way to ease into movement is to walk. It doesn't require any equipment other than a pair of shoes which I assume you have. Oh, and clothes. Please wear some clothes when you go out for a walk. This will prevent you from getting arrested.

You might still be stressed or ruminating or worrying while you're walking so I suggest bringing some favorite music to accompany you.[6] Walking also makes a great moving meditation; you don't need to sit still to meditate. In fact, this works much better for some people and is a great introduction to it.

All you need to do is focus on something other than your thoughts like your breath or the movement of your body.

You can also direct your attention to the things you see and hear. I guarantee you will find yourself wrapped up in your thoughts again and again (and again). That's okay, it's what happens during meditation for most of us. It's like a practice in directing your attention to the present and at first you won't be very good at it.

You're doing fine though just as long as you keep walking. Not forever though, as tempting as it may be, you might want to come back home and get some lunch.

---

6   Some people experiencing grief, depression, or anxiety feel repulsed by music and have no desire to listen to it. If this is you, note that your feelings are not abnormal, and that needing silence is absolutely okay.

Generate ideas

The brain, like other parts of our bodies, atrophies if it's not exercised. You could rush out and pick up the latest digital brain gadget or subscribe to expensive online programs but really all you need is a pen and paper. The instructions are simple: pick an issue or topic and try to come up with about 10 solutions or alternatives. It could be 10 ways to get out of debt, or 8 unrealistic careers you'd like to have or 23 different things you can do with a paper clip. There's no need for it to be serious or even practical, the best ideas often arise from the far edge of sanity.

Even if most of your ideas are lousy it doesn't matter, no one will know about them but you. It's the exercise that counts.

This very book is an example of a challenge I set for myself. I was lying in bed, grasping at the sleep that had eluded me for so long when I finally rolled out of bed at 3:00 am and was inspired to create this list.

I figured it would be a major challenge to generate 100 of anything so I kept my expectations low. It took about four days to reach my target. Then I kept coming up with more ideas. It was ridiculous. Ideas are akin to bacteria, duplicating like crazy until the entire human race is wiped out and all the animals rejoice. I think this is a good problem to have.

10

Call an old friend

This can be challenging or even embarrassing, especially when you kept meaning to call that friend, but it's been so long you keep putting it off because it's been so long that eventually years go by and you still haven't reached out and now you feel like a total heel. There's no way you could call now!

But there is. You just pick up the phone and dial. Or send an e-mail but calling is probably better. Do it quickly without dreaming up all the horrible things they might say because most of it is unlikely and even if they are angry with you, so what? Now you can stop thinking of calling that friend every twelve days or so and drop the guilt.

They'll probably be glad you had the courage to reach out to them.

11

Ask for help

Probably not someone you owe money to, but anyone else will do. Family, friends or strangers are all possible candidates. I've been surprised many times by what strangers will do for one another without the expectation of payback. Asking a stranger or acquaintance for help doesn't come with the baggage family and friends sometimes bring to the occasion.

You can ask for someone's listening, ask them to join you in an arduous task, ask them to keep you on track in reaching your goals. You can ask for support, or to look after your kid for a few hours.

The key to asking is deciding that you can accept "no" as a response. Even if it comes in the form of, "Oh, I'd love to babysit sometime! But gosh, it's just so busy and stressful being a single travel blogger, you know? She's so cute though, maybe when she's three?"

Sometimes you can't suppress an eyeroll. Just let that crap out.

12

Ask for professional help

If, like me, you have trouble asking for help then asking for professional help can be a daunting task to avoid for weeks, months, years even. It's hard to admit when we need help. There exists an unspoken code that we should be able to help ourselves, to stand on our own. We take pride in our independence. We would rather suffer indefinitely than ask for something we truly need.

In some cases, we may not even realize we need help.

Suffering and struggling to get through the day are not sexy. It's not a sign of your grit and determination. Why take the hard road when there are other options?

There is no glory in stoicism when it comes to your mental well-being and you're not fooling anyone around you.

If you can't do it for yourself then consider doing it for the sake of your loved ones.

13

Spend time with puppies

There is no way you can sit on the floor, surrounded by hyper bundles of fur and not feel fantastic. Puppies are a seriously neglected form of therapy. However, they can be addictive and should come with a...

WARNING:

Although you may derive delirious joy from being in the proximity of so much cuteness, do not give in to the temptation to take one (or three) home with you. Puppies, although adorable, require extensive care and training and in a short period of time become not-puppies. These delightful creatures will likely pee on your floor, eat your sofa, shed profusely, tear apart the garbage daily and roll around in poo. (And despite all this it's still easier to manage than looking after a baby.)

If you are prepared for the responsibility and pleasure of owning a pet, then by all means bring a dog into your life. As a fellow dog owner, I can attest to the joy and frustration of being a pet guardian. However, if you want to enjoy all the fun without the hassle just find a pup or three to hang with for a while.

14

Watch something funny

If you're already eroding months of your life watching YouTube videos, then you may want to consider picking a different medium to change things up. Otherwise, getting some laughs in is far better than lying in bed with a little rain cloud hanging over your head. I think I just wrote that because it's pouring rain today and I'm stuck inside. Which makes me think that it would be a prime opportunity to watch Dodgeball.

Bonus points for this one if you can find something funny to watch related to parenting. There are a few comedians who do justice to the topic like Michael McIntyre, Lisa Alvarado, Hugh Fink and Mary Ellen Hooper. Jim Gaffigan, father of five, has some zingy one-liners too:

"You want to know what it's like having a fourth kid?

Imagine you're drowning and someone hands you a baby."[7]

---

7   "Jim Gaffigan: Mr. Universe 2012." Accessed February 9, 2021 at https://www.quotes.net/mquote/1024890.

"Raising kids may be a thankless job with ridiculous hours, but at least the pay sucks."[8]

8   Jim Gaffigan. "Dad Is Fat", p.46, 2013 Crown Archetype. Accessed February 9, 2021 at https://www.azquotes.com/quote/625224.

15

Read fiction

A self-explanatory idea. For me the point is to escape my drab little life for a while and when I'm really down the lighter the fiction, the better. Why read dark, depressing stories when you're already hanging by a thread? I've made that mistake too many times and suffered too many sleepless nights as a result.

I recommend something funny, feel-good or sexy. Any of those themes are bound to draw you out of your current state. Ha "bound" wasn't even intentional, I swear. Although my terrible, pun doesn't really make a lot of sense if you're reading eBooks, unfortunately.

Give yourself a break, put down that self-help book and replace it with something more amusing. Even if it's this book.

16

Get lost

The strange thing about getting lost is it's easy to do when it's unintentional and hard to do when it's intentional. Every time I try to get lost, I find myself walking down a familiar street again. I tried this in London a few years ago and I couldn't seem to get away from Oxford Street. Everywhere I went bloody Oxford Street would pop up again. I felt like a flesh and bone boomerang. To fix this problem I hopped on a random double decker bus. A few minutes later I found myself outside Hyde Park and a block away from the Victoria and Albert Museum which happily turned out to be one of my favorite spots in London.

You don't need to cross the ocean to get lost, it's possible to do in your own town, something I have accomplished by accident many times. Take a bus or a train to an unfamiliar neighborhood and wander around the side streets. If you realize at some point that your wallet is missing you've picked the wrong neighborhood.

Even better, bring some people with you. It's much easier to get lost when everyone is arguing where to go.

17

Hello my name is...

Adding isolation to PPD is a toxic brew. It's too bad meeting new people with a child in tow can be a monumental challenge. Sometimes people click in a magical way and when that happens it's a golden moment. However, it usually takes a lot of time and patience. I've moved so many times that the pain of starting over has become a familiar friend.

The best way to meet people is to find others going through similar challenges. Our ability to bond seems to be enhanced in the context of strife.

I spent months trying to fit in with the members of a new mother's Meetup group in my neighborhood and through the local mom and baby playtimes at a community center. But it was hard to relate to the other parents who weren't experiencing PPD and I felt like a fraud in new mother's clothing (yoga pants and a t-shirt).

When I found a therapy group for mothers with PPD everything shifted. I was able to be honest about what I thought and how I felt while being surrounded by a chorus of nodding heads instead of judgements and scorn. Sometimes you need to step outside the safe bubble of home. Especially, when in crisis, you need an army of sisters who get you.

Even if you don't have access to a group like this where you live there are a number of online gathering places to vent or just revel in the familiar experiences of other distressed parents.

If you can't find any place online to settle in at least know that you are not alone because you have me and the words on these pages.

18

Do something you've never done before

Relax, I'm not going to suggest you try swimming with the sharks—just yet. Unless you want to. It could be something minor, like a gateway activity that leads you to bigger badass stuff you've never done before. I'm trying to think of some small thing I've never done before but it's five in the morning so I'm still a bit foggy and longing to crawl back under the covers.

One thing I had never done before was finish any of the major writing projects I'd started. With this book I decided to change that. Clearly, it's not an epic, 600-page paperweight but it took a lot of determination to keep writing when I'd rather be in bed reading things other people have written. At the time of writing this I was 83% complete (I didn't write each idea in order)—a significant accomplishment for me.

I suppose completing a book is a bad example of a minor thing I've never done before. As a natural-born introvert, going to any party with more than three people fits the definition of "badass" for me. You can take my sad example and improve upon it, I dare you.

19

Help someone else

Draw yourself out of your own misery and dive into someone else's! Helping other people is a nice diversion so long as you follow a few simple rules:

It's a good idea to make sure the person you intend to help actually needs and wants your help. Jumping in to help where it's not wanted is awkward and unfulfilling. I speak from experience.

You also want to ensure that you actually have the skill and capacity to help. No point in making things worse, that will only make you feel like a failure. And you don't need more of that right now.

Finally, in order to maintain your own sanity, set clear boundaries around your offer to help. This ensures the other person doesn't end up taking advantage of you or you overextend yourself voluntarily, whereby you go from feeling like an important and integral member of society to a bitter do-gooder.

Despite all these notes of caution, helping others is a great way to shift our focus from the daily slog of parenting with PPD.

20

Try a simple meditation

This meditation business seems daunting doesn't it? I mean, who is actually good at it? Certainly not me. Most of us won't be walking around with empty minds at any point in our lives so I think this is one area where it's very helpful to be realistic.

Just like the formation of life, start with itty-bitty goals like bringing your focus to your breath for one-minute, or counting breaths backwards from 20. By chipping off a small piece like this, even the most hyper mind could (potentially) achieve monk-like bliss.

Each time you find your mind wandering simply return your focus to the breath. There's no need to berate your brain for doing what it was designed to do—wander.

Another option is to repeat some kind of mantra (a short phrase) for one minute, the way Bart Simpson writes his lines on the chalkboard at the start of every episode. Only it might be best to keep the mantra short and positive. You can make one up, find one somewhere or just mentally chant OM.

Here are a few suggestions:

- I am peace. I am calm.

- Breathe in light. Exhale darkness.

- Grant me peace, strength, & courage.

21

Write

Are you worried that you suck at writing? That's okay, I often think I suck at writing too but that doesn't stop me. Well to be fair, sometimes it does. I occasionally become afflicted with a disabling disorder called procrastination. Thankfully, scientists have developed a simple cure. It involves... writing anyway. Yes, even if you don't feel like it.

Writing need not be brilliant, poetic or profound. It need not even be entertaining if no one else will ever read it.

In fact, you might not want to re-read your mangled masterpiece and that's great. Just write anyway. Put onto screen or paper whatever you want. A good place to start is to pick a topic or search online for "writing topics" where you'll find endless lists of ideas to unleash the Margaret Atwood that resides deep inside you.

Avoid getting hung up on spelling, grammar, or making sense. The best writing I've ever done was absolute nonsense which then became this book.

Create something

The act of making something beautiful where nothing existed before is the definition of creativity. A degree in fine art is not required in order to be creative. You can create art out of yarn or a bookshelf with scraps of wood in the garage. You can create a romantic dinner at your kitchen table or a park bench. You can create harmony with music or between co-workers where there was only tension before. You can create poetry or write elegant code or rebuild a bike out of donated scraps.

If you can't think of anything else to do just create some quiet time for yourself.

23

Do stuff with your non-dominant hand

If you are already ambidextrous, good for you. For everyone else, this is a simple, but not easy way to awaken some dormant cells in neglected parts of your brain. It really does make things different, not necessarily better, however. If you brush your teeth with your non-dominant hand, you'll probably do a pretty crappy job but think of all the new neural pathways you're generating!

There are lots of other fun things to try like putting your pants and socks on the other leg/foot first. I bet you didn't even realize you always put one particular leg in first, did you?

Wait... I feel a personal anecdote coming on...

In college I studied Graphic Design and Illustration. I'm terrible at drawing and I hate it. My Fourth-Year illustration teacher hated me too. He once told me that the drawings in my book were the kind of stuff we were doing in First Year. I wanted to punch him. We were forced to submit sketch books every quarter and were expected to fill them.

This is actually much worse than it seems. It was agony for those of us who despised sketching. We would panic and start filling our books two days before they were due.

Halfway through my final year I was failing illustration and I needed the course to graduate. One late night, a few days before sketchbook D-day, I was sitting in my room fuming over the harsh words from my instructor when I decided to unleash my contrarian trickster and draw with my non-dominant hand (which would be my left). I used a few magazine photos as inspiration since I suck terribly at life drawing (at which point you might wonder why I was in art college in the first place). I scratched out a few drawings and was relieved to have at least put in a good effort.

The next day I nervously handed my book to my nemesis, the illustration teacher. He looked at a few drawings and asked, "What's going on here? This is quite different from your other work."

I told him about my deviation. "I figured my drawing couldn't get any worse," I said.

"This is brilliant! Why didn't you start doing this earlier?"

Later that year I passed illustration and graduated with a degree in Visual Communications. I haven't touched a sketchbook since.

24

Quit something

Is there a commitment you've made that haunts you daily? Was there something you said "yes" to that you now deeply regret? If so, you may just want to quit. Free up some of your time for more delightful and spontaneous things. There is no shame in quitting unless you let the shame take over you.

Other people, who are threatened by your courage, will try to guilt you into staying. They are not the boss of you!

That could be your mantra, even. It's better if you don't say this out loud to them because it will make you appear juvenile. Try creating something intelligent and mature to say in response or, if you don't succeed, just smile and walk away or hang up the phone. The smiling is the important part, it will make you feel better.

You could also pull the politician card and say you're leaving to spend more time with your family.

25

Hit something

For heaven's sake not a person, unless they are wearing padding and you're in a self-defense class. No kicking small, yappy dogs either as tempting as that may be.

Pillows and sofas are a good choice.

There's not really much else to say on the matter, I think the title (with some cautionary fine print) speaks for itself. You can also scream into soft objects; I find doing so to be quite therapeutic and more productive than screaming at my husband.

26

Dance

Even if you have no rhythm, even if you have no coordination or even if you don't enjoy it, dance anyway. Make stuff up, do the same move over and over again, start slow and warm up to full self-expression. Dance alone, dance with friends, dance with people you don't know. Try dance classes or some obscure style like contact dance.

I'm grateful to have had access to a weekly freestyle dance event. The DJs play a bizarre variety of music from classical to hip hop and the dancers are equally as diverse. Children, seniors, pro dancers and average people like me fill the floor with our eclectic styles. Some of us are very skilled and some people just stand in one place and groove a little. People get down on the floor, lift each other up, and fill the space with energy.

You don't need a lot of space to do your thing, I only want to point out that you don't really have any good excuses to not dance. I've danced with children and people in wheelchairs.

Dancing is just moving to music, even toddlers do it. You don't need to be good at it, you only need to put your heart into it.

27

Listen to your favorite music

Forget sad songs.

Oh, I know you love drowning yourself in miserable lyrics until you want to jump off a bridge but avoid the temptation to do it this one time. Choose something upbeat, uplifting or groovy. Listen to it loud enough that the thoughts in your head need to yell to get your attention. It's easier to ignore the nasty voices when you're steering wheel drumming or testing the acoustics in the shower.

28

Buy some flowers

I never think to buy flowers. This idea was inspired by my husband who has a habit of buying flowers to brighten up our living room. It's not a regular thing, he might pick up a bouquet a few times a year, but it's more than I've ever thought of doing.

Every time he comes home with some flowers and we put them in a vase on the kitchen table I think, "this is a really good idea, we should do this more often". And then I promptly forget. Use this note as inspiration to bring a little life into your living space.

Flowers always look great and smell lovely. That is until they die, and you leave them to rot and grow moldy in the vase. Which I typically do. Please avoid doing that, it's demoralizing.

Eat well

Eating well is a challenge for a sugar addict like me, but I always feel better for doing so. I'm no nutritionist but here are a few ideas that may help you improve your diet:

- Remove all the tempting garbage food from your kitchen (and bedroom or wherever you hide it). Just throw it out. Avoid the rationalization that it would be awful to let that food go to waste and consume it all before you start eating well. I have done this, and I assure you it's not worth it.

- Replace garbage food with other snacks that are much better for you. Nuts and seeds are a great alternative as are fruit and cut veggies with dip. If you are an instant food kind of person, healthy granola bars can work too.

- Cut up the veggies when you bring them home so they are ready for snacking or meal prep. Keep your healthy food in the front and center of your fridge and cupboard, so you can see them easily. This is where you will first look when you open the door and we typically grab the first convenient food we see. We are really simple animals.

- Plan meals in advance and purchase the food you need about every 5-7 days. This is the ideal timeframe for grocery shopping. When we shop more or less often, we tend to buy too little or too much food and then forget what we bought.

Blend fruit and veggies into a smoothie so you can drink your vitamins and minerals. For some reason I'll eat well when I'm out but not so well at home. Liquid food has been my savior.

- Create a nutritionally balanced meal and eat that same thing every day for a few weeks or a month at a time. A few high achievers and crazy busy people I know use this technique. Of course, you need to prep a fresh batch every three days but it takes the planning and stress out of meals and ensures you're getting the nutrients you need so you can focus on other things.

30

Do one small thing each day

Big goals are daunting for most of us, especially a parent with PPD. A huge task is really nothing more than a compilation of little tasks that can be completed in a few minutes. Faced with a mountain of a project, get out your jackhammer and smash that baby into bite sized pieces. It's much easier to move mountains one stone at a time. It might take a while, especially if you have the Rockies in mind, but it's possible.

Pick a big, juicy goal or project that rests heavily on your shoulders, then think of one small task you can chip off today to get you started.

Pick another small task to complete this afternoon or tomorrow or this weekend. I find taking the first few steps to be the most challenging, but once I've set foot on the path, I can just keep walking, one foot in front of the other, until my son hits his head on something and starts screaming. Then I rush to him and completely forget what I was doing until I come across my half-finished project later that day where I will leave it to sit for a month until I get sick of looking at it or stepping over it. We all have our obstacles.

31

Drink enough water

Apparently, there has never been any research done to back up the eight glasses of water a day theory. However, don't let that deter you from getting enough clear fluids throughout the day. Quite often when we're feeling off, we reach for a snack when our body is really begging for hydration.

Water is essential to keep our metabolism functioning properly.[9] And yes, wine is "mostly water" but also has a dehydrating effect.

To prevent myself from forgetting to hydrate I keep a glass or water bottle always full and always within view. If I have a headache or I'm feeling sluggish a glass of water is often the cure. Yes, you will pee a lot in the early days, but your body will adjust. It's smart that way.

---

9   Joe Leech, "7 Science-Based Health Benefits of Drinking Enough Water." *Healthline*, (Healthline Media, June 4, 2017.) Accessed February 9, 2021 at https://www.healthline.com/nutrition/7-health-benefits-of-water.

Research a new career

Unless you are absolutely thrilled with your current career and your existing hobbies bring you endless joy, you might want to consider discovering what else is out there.

I suspect there is something you've dreamed about doing that you haven't had the time/energy/money to explore.

There are a few reasons why I highly recommend doing a little fieldwork: First, if you're not happy with your current occupation consider this your kick in the butt to take the first step toward a new career. Second, even if you enjoy your job but are lacking fulfillment in that area or in your life outside of work it could be that you need the right hobby or side project to light you up and energize you. There's no need to absolutely LOVE your job, it is possible to have a mediocre career that provides the funds for an inspiring hobby, one that keeps you happy and motivated full-time. Third, you may discover that it's not as difficult as you thought to make a sideways career move. Or you might find that although it will take considerable time and energy, it is manageable and possible to make a living doing what you've dreamed of while you stew in boredom at your current job.

And the final reason I recommend researching a new career is to find out if it's something you wouldn't like anyway so you can stop dreaming about it. This happened to me, having dreamed about being an architect since childhood. Now I'm relieved I didn't choose that path. The hours are long, the pay is terrible and unless you're a star performer at a prestigious firm, the work is boring. Plus, projects tend to have a lifespan of two years or more which far exceeds the limitations of my ability to focus. In other words, I would be a suicidal architect, so I enjoy the industry from afar and use it as an inspiration for my creative work.

In order to fully comprehend the effect a career change might have I recommend interviewing a number of people who do what it is you've dreamed of to get the most accurate picture of your new potential lifestyle. Visit them at work, see them in action, breathe in the aroma of your new career to find out if it's everything you imagined it would be. The last thing you want to do is spend years making that big move only to find out it's worse than your current job.

33

Be silly

I think we expend a lot of energy trying to look good. In reality, we are all weird. But it's the weird in us that makes us interesting. Then there are those who take weird to the extreme and actually wear it. In public. Like a costume. Don't be fooled by this phony freakishness. Trying to look interesting is the other side of the same coin that is trying to look normal. All you need to do is occasionally drop the normal act and just say what you really want to say or wear what you really want to wear.

This is challenging, I know. When you spend a long time pretending, it's hard to even know what or who you are. This can be compounded by the out-of-body experience of having a child and the permanent physical and emotional transformation that comes with it. This is why I recommend being silly, it's like practicing being real again by putting your restrained identity aside.

Learning to be yourself again is like any other kind of education. Start in small, private ways and work yourself up to public acts of absurdity. Just admitting to yourself alone how you might talk, walk or just be if you were being your honest self is a good start. Be intentionally strange in your living room when no one is around. Skip down the sidewalk in some foreign neighborhood. Talk to animals in the park or hug a tree when you think no one is looking. I don't know what being silly looks like to you. Maybe silly is wearing socks that don't match or donning superman undies beneath a tailored suit.

If possible, be silly with children. You won't look out of place and they'll love it.

Paint a room

Color has a profound effect on our mood, whether we notice it or not.

For the color obsessed like me it's a life and death thing. My spirit soars or dies according to the colors of the room I'm in so when it comes to my living space it's got to be filled with colors that I adore.

Even if you're not so attached to the hue of your bedroom your subconscious certainly is. Change up your space by painting the walls of one room (or even one wall) a new color. If you bomb on the color selection, it's no big deal to paint over it again. And if you've been wanting to repaint the walls and cupboards in your 80's inspired kitchen then what have you been waiting for? At worst it will take a weekend or so to accomplish. Paint is probably the cheapest way to quickly overhaul any space and a lot easier to alter if you make a mistake.

35

Rearrange your space

Some of us are very resistant to change. I seem to thrive on it. I've moved so many times that I start to get the itch to live somewhere new after a year of being in the same place. Instead of packing it all in, I've found it's far less stressful to simply refresh the space I'm currently in by rearranging the furniture.

Where you have your bed or your sofa right now might not be optimal, or it might be perfect. It's hard to tell unless you try a different setup. If moving big pieces of furniture is too daunting, then move around a few smaller pieces or rearrange the interior of a cupboard. While you're playing around you might find things you didn't know you had or thought you'd lost or wondered why you've been holding on to such a useless thing.

If you don't like the new arrangement, change it back.

36

Breathe

Sigh, this whole breathing business has become a cliché and yet it's so essential to our survival that you'd think we'd have the activity perfected by now. We forget to breathe when it's most critical to get oxygen to our brains so we can't think clearly in stressful situations. If our brain is oxygen deprived, how do we remember to do this? It's just like getting to Carnegie Hall—practice, practice, practice. The key is to train when your stress level is low and slowly work your way up just like learning to play the cello. Or learning anything, really.

It's hard to learn how to swim when you're drowning and the same goes for deep breathing.

I'm not even going to bother going over the basic steps like expanding the belly to pull air into the deepest part of the lungs and breathing through your nose, etc. If you didn't know how you were supposed to do it, you do now. Set up reminders to practice breathing a few times per day. Or, use your environment to act as a cue. When your child is eating or finally falls asleep, that could be a good time to slow down and focus on your breath.

As a bonus, all of our cells require oxygen to function and deep breathing sessions a few times per week help to super-oxygenate the cells. This keeps us functioning at our best and prevents aging, illness, anxiety and has too many other benefits to list.[10] Some people swear it prevents cancer, but they say that about a lot of things. I'll let you decide on that one.

---

10   Relaxation Techniques: Breath Control Helps Quell Errant Stress Response - Harvard Health." Harvard Health Blog. (Harvard Health Publishing, April 13, 2018.) Accessed March 12, 2020 at https://www.health.harvard.edu/mind-and-mood/relaxation-techniques-breath-control-helps-quell-errant-stress-response.

37

Stop listening to self-help gurus

Even if you think your ego might swell out of control without the daily wisdom of Eckhart Tolle, I encourage you to let him go for a while. A week, a month, forever, the timing is up to you. Stop fixing yourself, stop stressing out about your "pain-body" and take a break. There's probably nothing wrong with you anyway.

This goes for "baby-gurus" too. Sometimes all the knowledge you need is already inside you.

38

Clean

Dirty, messy spaces make my thoughts cluttered and muddy. And
I need all the clarity I can get. There are those who seem not to notice
the piles of laundry, receipts, and unopened mail tossed together on the
floor like a mixed salad. I'm married to one of those people. Having lived
in close proximity to a messy person for many years I believe that deep
down they really are bothered by the state of their clutter. Who doesn't
like a clean, tidy space? If given the choice would you not want to have
everything in its place, so you know where it is, but don't have to look
at it every morning and night?

I'd say it's not the state of being clean that bothers most of us, it's
the act of cleaning itself. We try to get comfortable with the scum in
the bathtub because it seems easier than putting on the gloves and
getting out the scrubby thing. But when my space has been cleaned and
polished and is looking its best, I feel better about the world.

The gleam, the open space, the breathing
room, is like therapy.

Until someone comes along and messes it
up again a few minutes later.

Tackle one small project that has been bugging you for ages

The longer I put off these kinds of things, the more gigantic and looming they become. Dumb little projects like returning an e-mail or making an important phone call weigh on me like a shirt made of lead. There's no good reason I have for not doing these things other than I don't feel like it. A smart friend once told me to stay away from those defeating words "feel like it".

When you're about to say to yourself that you don't feel like (or just after you've said them, which is what I do) consider saying something like, I'm going to do this thing right now and then reward myself by... [insert pleasurable activity here].

Tip number two comes from a book I started reading a few months ago. I still haven't finished it but there's a brilliant idea somewhere near the beginning that goes like this: If you get a thought to do something, act on it within 5 seconds or it will self-destruct. That's probably not what the author really wrote but that's how my little brain remembers it. This technique really does work, most of the time. I recommend giving it a try.

40

Brighten up your life

Dark spaces are a downer.

I once lived in an old house with small windows that felt gloomy even on the sunniest days. When we went looking for a new place, I had a firm requirement for big windows to let the sun in. If you don't have the option of renovating or moving, you can simply add more artificial light to your life. It's easy to find natural light bulbs with a decent wattage and thanks to LED or whatever new invention is popular at the time that you're reading this. It's also no longer a huge energy drain.

Spend time in nature

(Without music, without your phone, and without a flask of single malt scotch).

Take a few breaths of air that's been purified by the trees and shrubs around you. Listen to the subtle song of long grass moving in the breeze or the nails of a squirrel gripping the bark of a tree as she runs in terror from you. Really look at all the different kinds of plant life beneath your feet. It's not just a bunch of green stuff; there's a whole ecosystem there that will survive very nicely without us.

Even if you bring your offspring along and even if they are grumpy and not into this "bonding with nature thing", see if you can find the small spaces in their silence to capture the sound of the wind in the leaves.

As much as we try to avoid it, we are nature. Spend some time with your relatives, the ones who don't bicker and complain. The trees don't care if you forget to call, the bees don't care if you're late for work and the seagulls just want your lunch.

Enjoy.

Take a course

There's probably something you really want to do that you're not doing. I know what your excuses are, I've used them all. Maybe you think you'll fail, you can't afford it, or you don't have time. They all seem like really good reasons not to do something new, don't they? But really, they're lame excuses.

If you continued to peel away the layers of "reasons" you'd find something very vulnerable and tender. It could be something you don't want to face like the possibility of failure, the risk of embarrassment, the loss of your time or the dissolution of that dream.

Whatever it is you've always wanted to do, take one small step in that direction now.

Research the course you need then sign up. Find any activity in the vein of your interest that fits your schedule and your budget. When you make this kind of commitment delightful things start to unfold.

One of my passions is dance (I have many passions, unfortunately). But I have so many excuses for not committing to it more fully. I don't have the space to dance the way I want to; I live too far from the studio I want to train at. At one point I'd walked away from my previous career and had no money. I had a baby at home, I was out of shape (see the previous excuse) and I thought I'd look stupid because I'm probably not as good of a dancer as I think I am when no one is watching. That and I'd be older than everyone else.

For the past few years I've kept dreaming of some magical time in the future when I'll be a dancer. A time when I'll be able to perform on a stage and achieve great physical feats, leaving the audience in awe. I really just want to feel like I'm flying. But I have done nothing about this passion for so long that I'm going to be old and stiff if I keep up this pace. While I was working on this book, I received a flyer for a dance studio in the mail. It was near my house, it looked reputable, they taught some of the styles of dance that I love and that week they were accepting registrations.

A few days later I packed up my son (when he woke up from his nap) and drove over there to find out more about their courses. I was so nervous about taking the first step that I put off doing it the day before (babies are great excuses!).

In the end the studio didn't give me the right vibe and I decided against taking classes, but I'm proud of the initiative I'd shown at the time. I later became an aerialist, dancing in the air on silks or a hoop instead of on the ground. You never know what strange path you might end up on if you simply set one foot out on that journey.

43

Be spontaneous

I am a recovering planner. Having married someone who recoils at the prospect of planning I've begun to relax about needing to know how everything is going to play out before I begin. The other life change that has thrown a wrench in my perfectly laid out plans is having a kid. Children have a natural ability to completely derail any semblance of order your life may have had. All plans are off and as a parent, if you fight it, you usually lose. And then you get mad, and then you start thinking about how much easier your life was before and it's a dismal downward spiral.

Whether you live your life by a rigid routine, or you fly by the seat of your pants, be spontaneous in some way today. Do something that's not in your calendar, veer off your well-worn path to indulge in anything that grabs you.

Send kind notes to people you've neglected

There are those times when it's been too long since you've been in touch with someone that you put off contacting them because it's been too long, and they think you don't like them anymore or they did something to offend you, when really, you're just caught in the time/ fear circle and every day that passes just makes it worse.

For those times, send a note to say hello, I miss you, I really didn't forget about you, I'm just an insecure loser, etc. I'm not on a high horse here, I must certifiably be the absolute worst for this. It pains me to think about all the people I've neglected. Composing this idea has inspired me to send a note to someone. I highly recommend writing a silly book to inspire yourself. It's pretty neat. Or just write a note, which is a lot faster.

Hug someone

Really good hugs are golden. Some people have a natural talent for dispensing great hugs. I don't know exactly what the secret formula is, but I suspect it has more to do with wrapping love and joy around someone else. Maybe it's like a brief meditation where all you focus on is the hug itself. Not in that brief, awkward hug kind of way where you try to ensure very little of your body actually comes in contact with the other person. Those superficial hugs just don't make anyone feel good. Great huggers really commit to the embrace.

Pick someone, even your dog or cat, to really wrap your arms around and allow yourself to take a slow breath and make real contact with the other person (or pet). If you're feeling brave, try this suggestion I read somewhere many years ago:

When you hug someone,
be the last to let go.

XOXO

Talk to strangers

People in big cities can just ignore this bit of advice, they won't listen to it anyway. Being an introvert I'm not the most outgoing individual but when I first moved to Toronto from Calgary the cold, mega-city shoulder left me dumbfounded. I would stroll through High Park and as other people would pass by, I'd offer up a "hello" or "good morning", as one would typically do out West. But here, people avert their eyes or put their heads down and scurry along as if I were walking around in plaid pajamas with tinfoil on my head. It took me a few weeks to figure out that's not how things are done in the East. Unless you live on the outskirts of the Big Smog. Then you have to greet people, or they think you're an arrogant ass from downtown. And they'd sort of be right. How is a person supposed to keep track of all these varied social conventions?

I've devised a simple strategy; just talk to strangers anyway. So, they look at you like you're a crazy person who must be from Cowtown. In all likelihood you are a crazy person. If you really want to break the ice with ease bring along a dog or a baby. For some reason, no one here is threatened by a carnivore on a leash or a screaming person with a dirty pacifier.

Give something

(Anything but advice)[11]

Here is a list of things that are usually well received:

- Time. In person, or over the phone or in some other capacity.

- Listening. Really listening, not pretending and not waiting for your turn to speak.

- Blood. Costs nothing and can save the life of someone you will never meet. Plus, you'll get to find out your blood type, because I know you always wanted to know that.

- Old stuff you no longer need.

- Cookies, muffins or cake. Most people like one of those things. If not, they are weird or wheat intolerant.

- Energy. Help someone move, hang pictures, mow their lawn or some other activity that requires strength and vigor.

- Space. Especially if they ask for it. Really, they mean it.

- A smile or a warm gesture. It's free and makes you feel better too.

- Encouragement. We could all use a bit of that.

- I realize I haven't exhausted all the possibilities so go ahead and create your own gifts.

---

11   I am using this footnote to remind you that the items in this book are not advice they are *ideas*.

48

Receive a foot massage

No passionate lover required. Although it is nice to receive a foot massage from someone else (who knows what they're doing) you can also hit those reflex points on your own. All you need is a ball. That's it. Some of them work better than others and different kinds will deliver different results.

My personal favorite is a small foot massage ball with nubby bits all over it that provides an aggressive massage.

Another option is the squishy foam stress balls for which you will pay an absurd amount of money at some holistic store. As an alternative you could look for one of those blue, red and white ones at a dollar store. With the foam ball you simply need to stand on it and mash it under your foot.

As an experiment; look in the mirror before you begin to see where your shoulders are sitting. Mash the ball under one foot for about three to five minutes (or whatever you can spare between feeding or crying sessions) and look in the mirror again. You may notice the shoulder of the corresponding foot is now sitting lower than the other one thanks to this simple tension release. Complete on the other side to prevent lopsidedness.

Blow up your stress

Even if this doesn't eliminate your stress it's fun anyway. The only tool you need is a balloon, or a whole bag of them depending on how stressed you are.

Sit in a comfortable place, close your eyes and think about one worrisome thing. Concentrate on how you feel about it, where the stress resides in your body, notice your breathing change as you dwell on this lousy thing that's got you grinding your teeth as you sleep.

When you're ready, take a deep breath in and as you breathe out into the balloon, let your worry leave with your breath and fill the balloon. Keep filling the balloon with air and stress until you are lightheaded, or the balloon is fairly full. Tie the bottom, place it on the floor or hold it in your hands and pop it.[12]

Goodbye crappy, stressful thing. Repeat as needed.

---

12 Don't do this when your child has finally fallen asleep after two hours of coaxing.

50

Stretch

Most of us hold our stress in our bodies. We store our tension in two main areas, the shoulders (bearing the weight of the world) and our hips (I have no metaphor for this). The muscles are all connected in some way and stiffness in one area can affect other parts of the body as well. There must be a good reason why cats and dogs stretch continuously throughout the day, they certainly seem a lot more relaxed than most of us. Of course, they don't have bills to pay.

Whether you're a golden retriever or a cubicle dweller, stretching feels good, releases tension, and keeps the body in good form.

Have a look online or at the library for information on stretching depending on your situation. There are sets designed for people who sit at a desk all day and programs for beginners. You don't need to prep for Cirque du Soleil, just a few minutes per day will loosen you up. A flexible mind follows a flexible body.

Here are four quick muscle relaxers:

Shoulders: Shrug your shoulders and try to touch your ears. Squeeze for a moment before you breathe out and relax back down. Do this a few times until you feel your shoulders sitting lower than they were before.

Hips: Stand with your feet about hip width apart and your hands on your hips. Rotate your hips in a large circle in one direction about four to six times. Repeat in the other direction. Be sure to go through the full range of motion. If you notice your circle skips a bit that's an area of tightness in your hips that needs a little extra attention.

Neck: Gently turn your head to the right and hold for a moment before turning to the left. Return to staring straight ahead. Tilt your head down and hold it, then tilt it back as far as is comfortable. Return to start. Tilt your head to the side so your ear is facing your shoulder. Repeat on the other side.

Full body: Standing in a comfortable position simply reach for the stars. Reach as high as you can, feeling all of the muscles in your body drawing upward toward the sky. Sometimes I like to do this with my hands clasped in order to stretch my sides more intensely. I'm a sucker for pain.

I'm sure you feel more relaxed just reading this.

51

Say goodbye

(To someone)

I have done this and it's hard, I won't sugar coat it.

Saying goodbye to a relationship that just isn't bringing the goods is absolutely worth it though. I had a "friend" who was always generating one crisis after another and leaning on me for support. At first, I found the drama thrilling, my life appeared sane and boring in comparison. I was far too responsible which apparently makes me a handy crutch for nutty people. After years of being a dutiful support system I figured she would turn her life around and blossom so I could bask in the good work I had done. But this never happened. And the drama went on for a few more years before I realized what an incredible thorn in my well-being this relationship was.

I put to work the tried and true method of avoiding her in the hopes she would get the message and fade away. It didn't work. Figuring out how to "solve" this relationship began to consume my thoughts.

How do you tell someone you don't want to be their friend anymore? It felt like the worst kind of breakup. Yet 6-year-old girls do this effortlessly, what's wrong with me?

I decided to write a letter (not an e-mail, an actual letter). My search online for gentle breakup letters was a complete bust. It seems the only people who want to end friendships are those who have been brutally wronged; I was just a jerk. Despite the anxiety I felt, I did my best and went out on my own, a pioneer in the land of breakups. To ensure she received it I sent it through registered mail which cost me a bit of coin, but it was cheaper than therapy. I haven't heard from her since.

Or, you could just take my sister's advice for getting rid of people: lend them money.

52

Early to bed

Some of us are true night owls and others are early risers. Then there are the mid-day people, a tribe of which I might be a member.

Finding the right time slot for yourself can deeply affect how awake and energetic you feel during the day. Experiment with different bedtimes for a week to see how it affects your sleep and your waking hours. It's best to get into bed at the same time each night and wake at the same time, according to every sleep expert I've come across and there have been many of them, I assure you.

If after a week of early bedtimes, you still feel like crap, you're probably a night owl. Don't fight it. If your sleep schedule is a disaster thanks to your child or other factors in your life, I encourage you to take the necessary steps to make your sleep a priority regardless of what your mother or the attachment parenting gurus say.

53

Take things one day/ minute at a time

When I'm exhausted and overwhelmed, I tend to dwell on the big picture and panic. A bird's eye view of life makes it appear as though there's too much stuff to cram into the few decades I have left. And yes, I realize that seems absurd but I'm not likely to become a breakdancing champion at the tender age of 80.

When I'm neck deep in worry, I have to remind myself to turn my focus to the minutes and seconds that make up the moments of my life before I go under. In those very small moments, there are no immediate concerns, there's a kettle boiling water for tea, a little boy who wants someone to read him a book and a dog that wants a belly rub. All very manageable things.

Once I've got my head out of the rainclouds, I'm able to decide what small step I'm going to take now to move forward. When I tell myself to just walk over to a certain spot and pick up one item I need, all the other steps begin to unfold like a domino train.

We each have 525,600 minutes in a year. That's a lot of opportunity to pull back from the race and refocus on our next steps or just savor our next breath.

Change your hair

You could shave it all off or get extensions but that might not be necessary. And, you might regret it.

But you could style it differently, color it, use a different hair product to hold it in place or put a wig on it.

For most of my adult life a ponytail was my go-to hairstyle. It's so ubiquitous that when my son illustrates his mother, she always has a dark blob on the back of her head.

"What's that on mommy's head, honey?" I ask.

"That's your ponytail!" he exclaims. It's both cute and depressing at the same time.

After realizing I was a one-trick-pony (ha) I went looking for simple alternatives online. I've found a few ideas that have worked well though many of them were far too complex for me to ever bother with (who has that kind of time in the morning?!) but at least I have two or three new styles in my arsenal.

55

Wear your best clothes

For no reason, other than because you want to look outstanding. When I (think) I look great this usually translates into feeling better about myself. When I feel like a bum, a pair of jogging pants rarely helps unless I actually go jogging, which I won't do because I can't get off the couch.

If you're like me, you have clothes you really love but never wear for fear you might ruin them. The idea of having something nice that just sits neatly in a drawer or draped on a hanger used to make sense to me. It was as though having a lovely article of clothing that I could wear if the occasion warranted it made the scrap of fabric seem like an object of worship. But usually, it ended up being a reminder that this mythical invitation from the Queen was not likely to occur. And even if it did, by the time it happened my precious item would be out of style.

I've now recovered from this wasteful, sentimental behavior and I sometimes reach into my closet and pull out something fabulous to wear on a Tuesday, for no reason, knowing that between the dog and the baby there is a good possibility that I will need to break out the stain remover.

56

Wear your PJs

There's a difference between feeling too lazy or depressed to get out of your PJs and intentionally going about your day in your nighttime attire. This idea was inspired by someone I'm married to who often goes for brunch on Sunday wearing what he slept in. Thankfully he does not sleep in the nude. Rather, he heads out in an old t-shirt and plaid flannel pants with an elastic waist that look absurd with pretty much any kind of footwear.

At first, I was embarrassed. But I've learned to embrace his laid-back approach and I too have worn my PJs to an all-day breakfast.

Since then I've noticed a few odd souls who dare to wear their PJs in public, usually to dine at a greasy spoon on a Sunday morning or to take the dog for a stroll through quiet neighborhood streets. As long as you've brushed your teeth and don't shout biblical quotes at stray cats or mutter conspiracy theories to yourself, you're OK.

57

Pick an interesting historical figure and read their biography

This suggestion may bring forth painful memories of history class, but I assure you this is way more fun. What? Fun? Yes. Because history is insane and stranger than fiction.

To begin with, you get to pick what you want to read, there are no deadlines, no essays or exams to write and no one who wants to steal your lunch money. I'm not much of a historian but the few biographies I have read have been fascinating. They are usually much juicier and entertaining than any history text I was forced to read in school.

If you're opposed to this idea you could even read some historical fiction, it's probably just as accurate. As Napoleon once said, "What is history, but a fable agreed upon?"[13] But then he also said, "Women are nothing but machines for producing children."[14] He's lucky I wasn't married to him.

---

13 The actual source of this quote is debatable. See: "What Is History But a Fable Agreed Upon?" Quote Investigator, 28 Mar. 2019. Accessed February 9, 2021 at quoteinvestigator.com/2016/07/05/fable/.

14 Napoleon Bonaparte, *The St. Helena Journal of General Baron Gourgaud, 1815-1818:* A Diary written at St. Helena during a part of Napoleon's Captivity, translated by Norman Edwards, 1932. Accessed February 9, 2021 at www.azquotes.com/quote/31298.

Make someone else look good

Doing this for another person is far easier than doing it for yourself.

Not only is it personally rewarding it can strengthen or improve a rocky relationship, especially at work. Of course, to expect some great karmic return would only lead to upset if it didn't happen so my advice is to leave your expectations of payback in your pocket. When you intentionally make other people look good, it's empowering for you because you own the circumstances you've just created. As opposed to someone else taking advantage of you in which they claim ownership. The outcome might appear the same, but I would say it's not—the prevailing emotions are entirely different.

You don't need to make a huge production out of it, making someone else look good can be as simple as a few key words delivered at the right time.

Give someone else credit and see what happens. It might not rain gold for you every time but when it does rain, it pours.

59

Do nothing

I find doing nothing kind of hard. I feel as though I should be making progress somewhere in my life, even if it's just picking yesterday's clothes up off the floor.

Some people excel at this without regret and I almost envy them.

There are lots of ways to do nothing, it does not require laying on the floor and staring at the ceiling for an hour. When someone is a jerk to you, decide to do nothing. Instead of making a big decision today, do nothing. If the dishes are piled high but there's a fiery, pink sunset on the horizon, don't wash a damn thing.

I could have used this today when I told myself I had to write. "Do nothing", my mind called to me, "set an example for the world", it rationalized. However, my looming deadline convinced me I could do nothing after I put a few words on the page. And that is what I'm going to do now...

60

Play with kid's toys

Any Lego fans out there over the age of twelve? You can't see, but my hand is in the air. I discovered how amusing toys can be when I started playing with my son's toys when he was a toddler. Maybe I'm just childish or maybe it really is therapeutic. At the very least the bright colors and obnoxious music will give you a new appreciation for peace and quiet.

Play any way you like, exercise the dormant parts of your brain by inventing as many different patterns as possible with a train set. Build a mediaeval castle out of Mega Blocks. If you don't mind the racket, get out some wooden spoons, pots, and pans to start your own kitchen band. Your neighbors will never forgive you.

61

Invite a friend over for a game

I hate playing games. That might be because I never play them so I'm not good at them, therefore I always lose which is a bit depressing. Pictionary would be the only exception. I'm pretty good at charades as well. Essentially, I'm awful at strategy games or those involving luck. Oh yeah, I also like solitaire but that doesn't count in this case because the point is to engage with friends and other loved ones.

Recently someone mentioned Twister—a game I'd long forgotten about but could be fun to play with someone you have a crush on. Or are married to which might spice things up a little.

If you've forgotten about games and left them to collect dust in a closet, this is a way to get out of your cave and interact with people you care about. You also get the benefit of mental exercise to tone up the parts of your brain that may have been neglected lately. I just need to keep reminding myself it's not about the win.

Tell someone how much they mean to you

This is harder than it sounds so don't think too much about it—just go for it.

Do it in writing or emojis if you must. As awkward as it may feel for you, most (normal) people very much appreciate being told that they mean a lot to someone else. It doesn't happen very often and that makes it all the more meaningful and memorable. You can't go wrong here, just keep it short and honest.

If the subject of your appreciation doesn't seem to be moved that's ok. They may simply be hiding their joy under a reserved façade or they may have been caught off guard. Regardless of the reaction you receive, understand that you did make a difference even if only for yourself.

63

Read the Velveteen Rabbit

There are times when a name or a book keeps popping up during my reading and eventually, I get the hint from the universe that I need to look further. This was the case with the Velveteen Rabbit. Apparently, most people read this in childhood, but I think I was in my early twenties when I discovered it.

All I need to say about this book is that I must have a box of tissue nearby before I even open it.

The story is elegant and moving to the point where just thinking about it changes the space I'm in. If you have not read it or if it's been ages since you have, it's time to (re)acquaint yourself with this remarkable book.

64

Say no

Stop doing things you don't want to do. Even if it's only for one day or one week or one hour. If, like me, you have a hard time saying "no", then you probably need to work that muscle. This is a common issue so no need to berate yourself over it. Many of us were trained at an early age to be agreeable. As children we may not have been allowed to have a voice and, even though we are no longer in the same circumstances, we behave as though the constraints are still there—like an invisible tether. We may find that "yes" escapes our lips before we've even understood what we're agreeing to.

Think of the word "no" as your ally. It's there to take care of you, to make sure your needs are met, to safeguard your sanity.

It need not be harsh or abrupt but that one little syllable may feel rough as it leaves your lips if you're not used to putting yourself first. Try saying it as a warm-up before you get out into the world and put that "no" into practice. This tiny word is the secret code to the freedom club.

65

Say yes

In an apparent contradiction to the previous concept I present to you, the "yes". These two are like sisters and not actually in disagreement, although siblings are known to have their differences. I feel the need to clarify the profound difference between saying "yes" to something you're afraid of and saying "yes" to something that's not good for you. The trick is to know the difference and only you can determine what you truly need.

When we sign up for something that draws us out of the comfortable life, we were trying our damndest to maintain, it can be frightening. I believe, each time we agree to take on something bold it should hurt a little—those are growing pains. As long as we continue to challenge ourselves the pain doesn't go away but rather becomes our companion, a reminder that we are not degrading into complacency. Like the pain after a good workout that lets us know our body is getting stronger, the feel-good ache of saying "yes" to adventure is our coach along the way.

I know I've made this whole "yes" thing seem rather masochistic but it's not like having your arm sawed off after taking only a swig of whisky. It's the internal flutter of excitement, a physical sensation identical to fear, only our mind determines if it's one or the other. So, choose to feel excited rather than alarmed.

Let me think about it

(Buy yourself time)

I have a terrible habit of saying "yes" most of the time. Even when people don't ask me for help, I jump in and attempt to solve their problems. It's draining, and I usually end up overbooking myself. Then I feel bad because I have to cancel, or I'm bitter because my mouth forced me to do something that I wasn't interested in doing to begin with.

Recently I've become fond of saying "let me think about it." It sounds simple and elegant but it's hard to remember to do when you're up against the wall. I probably don't use it as often as I ought to, but I'm learning—albeit the hard way.

There's no reason you have to give someone an answer right away and if they demand one, then run. You don't need to be under that kind of pressure. Even if you're sitting in the interrogation room from Law and Order, you don't have to say anything until your lawyer arrives. That's one of the important things I've learned from TV.

Taking a few minutes to process a request will help you determine if it's something you really want to agree to.

Give yourself a little space.

67

Try new food

Eat something today that you've never had before. A foreign cuisine offered at a shady looking place down the street, an odd-looking fruit in the grocery store or something someone made, and you can't quite tell what it is. The novel flavors swirling around in your mouth have the capacity to expand your palate and your mind. Even if you don't like it at least you don't have to wonder anymore. If you decide to stay the course, the strange new taste might grow on you. Besides, there are people who managed to acquire a taste for Brussels sprouts, tuna eyeballs or black salted licorice. In my opinion however, only crazy people eat the eyes of fish.[15]

---

15 A few years after writing this I fell in love with Brussel sprouts sautéed in oil with bacon.

68

Take a looong shower

In addition to long showers I also recommend acquiring a massaging showerhead. Trying to bathe with a sprinkle of water dripping on your head makes cleanliness a chore rather than a joy.

There are many benefits to a long shower. To begin with you can get clean and therefore not smell and we are all grateful for that. You can get some good thinking done while the fast-moving water emits negative ions that destroy free radicals. According to WebMD.com, negative ions react in our bodies to increase serotonin, a feel-good brain chemical.

A shower can make a great start to the day, even if you got up on the wrong side of the bed.

69

Get a white board for the bathroom

Do you achieve your most brilliant work on the throne? Only to have your toilet paper masterpiece rush down the drain as you flush? Then put that genius on a whiteboard! In the bathroom! Stash a mini board between the toilet and tub or hang it on the wall. It's a great place to store all the important ideas you came up with in the shower or while relaxing in the bath. Many of my friends are artists who like to doodle while they... you know.

I take pictures of our artwork before I erase it to reveal a blank canvas. I've used it to record to do items, things to buy, names of people I need to call or other remarkable insights I don't want to forget. It's fun, unusual, and useful.

70

Call a random person from your address book

Just open it up right now whether it's manual or digital. Point at a name and dial. If, like me, you never clean out your address book and it's full of names you don't recognize you can have a free pass and try again. Then make a note to clean out your address book. If you are feeling rather bold just call one of those unidentified people and figure out who in heaven's name they are.

I have no idea what you should say to them, they're not my acquaintance. As a suggestion you could try truthfully asking how they are doing with the intent to actually find out how they are doing. This habitual question isn't used at all in some countries. I discovered this when a friend of mine from Holland told me how impressed she was that everyone in Canada wanted to know how she was. So, she actually told them—in detail. Only to find out a few months later it was just a pointless formality.

If your address book is a disaster, as mine is, use this suggestion to clean it out instead.

71

As soon as you think of a person— call them

I know someone who does this and it's pretty cool despite me having a bit of a phone phobia. My fear is that I'll bother someone at a bad time, they won't want to hear from me, or they'll keep me on the phone for an hour. Despite my silly, deeply ingrained fear I still think this is a great idea.

Here's what he does: We're all sitting around having a drink or something and this guy, let's call him Eddie, is telling a crazy story about someone he used to work with. As soon as he finishes the story, he says something like, "man, I haven't talked to that guy in forever" and he just rings him up right there. Eddie tells the person he's calling that he was just thinking of him and telling the story about the time they, blah blah blah... you get the idea. The conversation lasts about 2-3 minutes tops and then Eddie is back in the conversation with us.

Maybe you have to be a certain kind of person to pull this off, but you could be that certain kind of person a few times in your life, no? Pick up the phone and call someone you were thinking of and tell them you were just thinking of them and wanted to say hi. Who doesn't like being thought of? Or, if you are really pressed for time, just send a text message. That works brilliantly too—especially for phone-phobes like me.

72

Send a postcard or a letter

Few people do this anymore. This is to your advantage because it can become a great way to leave an impression. I can't recall the last time I received a hand-written letter and I'd probably be apprehensive to start one myself considering there is no undo button. That might be why my preferred writing instrument is a pencil.

You could also send a postcard from wherever you are, even if you're at home, just to let someone know you're thinking of them. Postcards are like old school picture text messages. They're quick and to the point—great for people who don't have a lot to say or don't want to say too much. One February I sent out Hello Kitty Valentines to a handful of good friends. Aside from the challenge of collecting addresses it was easy and fun. As a bonus, I got a nice little thank you note from each person on my list.

73

Find a local waterfall

Even if it's only a foot high there must be some water falling from somewhere. Even if it's man-made, that counts too. The sound of rushing water alone can help to block out the obnoxious and excessive noise in your head or coming from the stroller in front of you. As a simple and quick meditation, focus on the natural white noise for as long as possible. When you realize your mind has begun to wander just repeat the process.

Just like taking a long shower, fast moving water in nature releases even more negative ions that provide you with another serotonin boosting opportunity.

So even if your mind is really racing, you'll reap at least one invisible benefit from your effort. Maybe that's the reason the little piles of rocks with water trickling through them are sold at so many dollar stores.

74

Go to a performance for a band you've never heard of

This could turn out to be a remarkable discovery or simply cause hearing loss. To avoid the latter, I suggest earplugs as basic insurance. Drag a friend or book along with you so you have someone to sit with at a café if the band turns out to be a bomb. This works best when the band is local or small and the performance is cheap or free.

I have discovered a few of my favorite bands and artists this way. I've also sat through a small number of dreadful auditory experiences but so far there hasn't been anything that prevented me from leaving except for the guilt inflicted upon me by the friend who was performing.

Have sex

(With yourself or someone else)

And if you're not into it, that's okay too.
No pressure.

76

Eat something you love

How could you go wrong with this? Oh wait, you could overindulge and then regret ever meeting that box of cinnamon Danish cookies, swearing out loud you will never touch another one so long as your heart keeps beating. Which might not be very long since the sugar rush could kill you.

Or you could be composed and reasonable and just eat two cookies. Very slowly, savoring each bite. Notice the rush of saliva as you breathe in the flavors before you even open your mouth. Feel the crunch and crumble as you bite down, make note of the texture with your tongue and enjoy the sweet icing followed by the spicy cinnamon. Let the treat linger in your mouth before you swallow, only to follow with another slow, savory bite.

This is how you truly enjoy food you love. So I've heard.

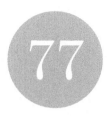

Write a song

Especially if you can't play an instrument or sing. I can hear your protests already:

I'm tone deaf (do you even know what that means?)

I have no rhythm (that might be true)

Um, I don't have a clue how to write a song (who does?)

That sounds hard (it's not)

I only sing when I'm drunk (go get a beer)

There are probably other variations of those excuses, but I think that sums it up. I'm not suggesting you try your hand at composing a chart-topping, multi-platinum single. That would be absurd because you probably don't have the marketing budget to pull it off regardless of whether or not you have talent. In fact, you don't even need a pencil to generate your very own snappy ballad, just steal one from someone else. Something timeless and catchy like Row, Row, Row Your Boat with new lyrics composed by you.

Okay, that sounds pretty simple, but what should you sing about? You could go on about whatever you're doing at the moment but the best topics to sing about are the things that bug you. Personally, I like to sing about how much my dog sheds. I don't think he really cares for my singing, but it does make me feel lighter when I'm wielding a sticky roller to get fur off the sofa.

You could sing about your ex, washing dishes, how painfully slow the cashiers are at Walmart, and so on.

For inspiration here's a little ditty my husband composed one morning when the sun was beating down on us through the skylight.

[Sung (badly) to the tune of *Tomorrow* by Annie]

The sun'll come out... right now
bet your bottom dollar that it will
The sun'll come out... right now
so you can't sleep in at all

The coffee, the coffee
I love you, the coffee
you're only a cup awaaaay

Oh, and did I mention the song need not make sense or be coherent? See, no pressure at all. Now go forth and compose, my newly minted maestro!

Here's one I just wrote that you can steal:

Twinkle twinkle
screaming child
life with you is really wild

Sometimes mommy wants to die
but then you smile
and I wonder why

twinkle twinkle
screaming child
I need to lay down for a while

78

Let go of success

I don't know what your definition of success is, but you might be better served if you let go of it. Even just for one day. It's probably unfounded and unrealistic anyway. Because, if it weren't, I doubt you'd be reading this book.

Consider that success does not occur when you have arrived somewhere, or you've made it to whatever standard you or someone else has arbitrarily set.

Those are merely the results. Success occurs when you are sitting in the blinding darkness of your lowest low and you draw up the courage to take another breath, to give it another day. That, in my experience, is one of the hardest things to do. If you can achieve that, you have found success.

Ask unusual questions

Ask friends, ask strangers, or ask yourself. Unconventional questions alter the kinds of conversations you'll have and what you'll learn about yourself and others. I'll admit I'm the kind of person who dreads small talk but engages in it anyway because I don't know what else to say. I've been inspired by friends and acquaintances who have a habit of asking unusual questions. Recently, I was reading a book where the author asked, "what was one of your favorite childhood memories?" The answer has been rolling around in my brain for days as I cobble together a collection of events from my childhood.

To help you out a little, here are a few of the great ice breakers I've encountered:

- What was one of the most embarrassing things that ever happened to you?

- Who were your childhood heroes?

- What superpower would you most want to have?

- Name one of your secret indulgences...

- Who is your famous crush?

- What was your favorite childhood toy?

- Do you like your name? And if not, what would you change it to?

- Where is one place you'd never want to visit?

- What is your favorite line from a movie?

- If your home burned to the ground, what three things, aside from your loved ones, would you save?

- What does the concept of a "soul" mean to you?

- When in your life did you feel most peaceful?

80

Fall in love

With anything, or anyone. Someone you may never meet, something you may never acquire. Love need not be reciprocated or expressed to the object of your adoration, but you can hang posters on your wall or wallpaper your desktop with its lovely image. It's okay to let yourself go, to feel the rush of the fall and just enjoy it. At some point you may fall out of love or move on. Just allow yourself to feel without trying to alter or rein in your emotions, a nearly impossible thing to do anyway.

If love feels like it's miles away from where you are now that's okay too. It happens, and it doesn't make you an awful person.

81

Want what you already have

There never seems to be enough. Perhaps it's a residual brain function to ensure our survival and it doesn't work so well in this current culture of abundance. At some point in our lives we truly wanted most of the things we have; with the exception of family gifts you've been emotionally blackmailed into keeping. Otherwise, most of the stuff was just a dream before you acquired it (including the people in your life). If you have things you don't want anymore, get rid of them. Otherwise, consider that you still want and adore what you already have. Those lovely things don't need to be replaced unless they are broken and not fixable.

If you are drawn to acquire new things, then stay away from places that tempt you. Recovering alcoholics don't browse liquor stores unless they want to relapse. I know how the game is played; I work in marketing.

Although the new-love high eventually fades there may still be some magic there. Get out your toolbox and make a few adjustments to get that relationship to your stuff working good as new.

82

See the gift in your struggle

What gift? Are you crazy? This sh*t that I'm going through right now sucks. Period.

When the going is tough, like marching through a muddy bog in the dark, it's hard to recognize the journey as anything but a lump of coal. When you stop just long enough to catch your breath there might be an opportunity to notice what this rough patch has to offer. There is some small glimmer of light no matter how dark of a place you're in now.

As I struggled with being a new parent I realized (eventually) that the challenges I faced made me far less judgmental of others. Not just other parents but anyone whose shoes I haven't walked in. Which is pretty much every other person who ever lived. I'm also learning to be less critical of myself. That last part is a little harder— we're always the most judgmental of ourselves—and it's not exactly helpful.

You don't need to do this right now, but at some point, it will become clear that there is a strange gift, however small, in the battles you're currently fighting.

83

Give some more

When it feels like every ounce of energy has been drawn out of you, when you think your next move is to the street—there is a chance to give. But how can you give when you feel like you've got nothing left?

There is always something you have to offer; this is how you get paid in the future. You do your part and the universe responds (eventually). I don't know why this little bit of magic works but let's just go with it.

I was really broke a few years ago. Broke to the point of not knowing how I was going to pay my rent in a few weeks. It was scary, I'd already exhausted my savings a while back. Such is the nature of being self-employed.

For some reason I decided it would be better to do anything at all than to sit around my apartment dreaming of being homeless. It was easy to narrow down my options, I had no money, and lots of time. It also occurred to me that I was in good health, something to be grateful for. So, I decided to give blood and get some cookies for my effort.

The actual bloodletting was a harrowing experience (I'll spare you the details) and I was glad when the whole thing was over, but I still felt good about my contribution. I was also informed of my blood type which, ironically, is B positive. Oh yeah, and they didn't have any cookies, I think it was granola bars or something as equally disappointing.

Now that I'd done my good deed you're waiting for the part where the universe gives back, right? Well, the big milky way did not disappoint. A few days later a friend called to ask if I wanted to help paint a big house they had just bought to flip, and they wanted to pay me for my effort. I was working as a designer at the time, but I know how to wield a brush, so I agreed. That month I didn't end up on the street.

Now I can't guarantee that you will be rewarded within the week, sometimes giving takes a little longer to boomerang but if you just keep giving out as much as you can, the universe will reciprocate, often in unexpected ways.

84

Memorize something

Here's something that I've memorized from the Tao Te Ching:

"What is of all things most yielding, can overwhelm that which is of all things most hard. Being substanceless it can enter even where there is no space." [16]

Although, to be fair, what I memorized is some guy's English translation of that bit of wisdom from the Tao Te Ching.

The answer, by the way, is *water*. What Lao Tzu is trying to say in a really complicated way is that we should aspire to be like water, moving smoothly and swiftly, wearing down the hard, unmoving rocks. It's pretty much the only thing I've ever memorized, and I use it to impress people. Aren't you impressed?

There is a point to memorizing something. For me it's a healthy distraction from the rattling noise in my brain. It can also serve as a reminder of something important that you want to remember, something that guides you. Or it can just cheer you up like a quote from someone who makes you laugh. I have a bunch of those, I just can't recall any of them right now.

---

16 Lao Tzú, *Tao Te Ching*. (Wordsworth Editions, May 7, 1996), p. 46.

Do something weird

(In public)

There are a lot of things that aren't illegal but aren't socially acceptable in public. We often don't think much about the social rules we were raised with and it can be liberating to challenge those concepts.

What if you were to just lie down for a rest in a public place? When you consider how bizarre this would look or how uncomfortable it would be both physically and socially it seems unappealing—especially to me. I haven't tried it yet; I'm worried people will rush over and think there's a medical emergency. To combat this and to make this idea a little more appealing, try being weird with a friend. It's not as risky but is more of a steppingstone toward braver, more exciting things.

You could also dress up in a costume and ride the bus, or dance on the sidewalk by yourself, or whatever else you can think of that scares the pants off of you. Like maybe bottle feeding in public.[17]

---

17   That was my own thing that I still haven't gotten over to this day.

Everything is better by candlelight

Feel as though you look haggard or maybe your space is a dust covered disaster?

The answer is candlelight.

The warm, gentle light of a candle makes everything look and feel romantic and dreamy, even your exhausted self, eating a bowl of mac & cheese direct from the pot. Candles alter the mood of your environment and the mood in your head. The light is easy on the eyes and many people meditate by gazing into a flickering flame. It's a pretty nice way to ease into a state of flow and great for people who tend to lack focus.

For the healthiest outcome I recommend beeswax candles but if the price tag freaks you out, soy or another vegetable-based wax is a good choice. Anything but paraffin. Apparently, it's flaming death. Oh, and look for a wick sans lead. I think everyone now knows breathing in lead is a bad idea.

Of course, the battery models are decent too and less of a hazard with children.

87

Take extra good care of yourself

Vitamins, floss, sunscreen, apple a day—aren't you worth taking care of? Even for an hour or just three minutes, pamper yourself with goodness. Be a slightly better you for a while, even if it's only one thing like being on time or getting out of bed a little earlier. It doesn't have to be a lifelong commitment but if it works for you consider keeping your new habit.

No pressure from me or from yourself to overhaul your life. This is but a wee experiment.

88

Sleep in

All the sleep experts say you're not supposed to change your sleep schedule because it will cause you to shrink 12 inches and grow two heads and so on. But what's wrong with one good lay in bed all morning as a special treat? You don't even have to sleep, just lie there all snuggly in the covers and daydream about the boring, productive things you could be doing that require work and effort.

Of course, if you're slave to a child, that might not be possible but see if you can arrange for it once-in-a-while.

Even if you have a lie-in with your babe while they eat breakfast everything is better in the womb of your bed.

89

Go slow

I don't mean move in slow motion. But that could be fun too, especially at work. Maybe you'll be more productive? I'm inspired here by the book *In Praise of Slow* by Carl Honoré.[18] He's an excellent writer and it's an intriguing idea. I can be hyper and impatient at times and when someone gets in my way (I'm looking at you, slow drivers) I get angry. It's an awful downward spiral.

In order to slow my pace, I first remember to breathe. And then I remind myself that I'll get there when I get there and being a minute earlier is not worth the stress or the potential whiplash.

When it comes to eating, I shove food in my mouth like it's the dinner Olympics. I'm probably a record holder. In my defense I inherited the speed eating gene from my father. Or maybe it was learned. Either way, I know I have control over how quickly I polish off my tuna melt, I just don't choose to exercise that control. You shouldn't use me as an example of how to go slow, I'm terrible at it.

Instead, read Carl's book or find an excerpt online. It might inspire you to turn the dial down.

---

18   Carl Honoré. In Praise of Slow: How a Worldwide Movement Is Challenging the Cult of Speed. (Seven Dials, 2019.)

90

Stop explaining

"Explaining is draining"[19]
- James Altucher

This is an idea I like to put into practice but often forget. It's a habit of mine to provide more information than necessary and it bugs me. When I think of the amount of time that I've wasted explaining my actions when a few simple words would have sufficed I've probably lost a few months of my life, maybe more.

In most situations you don't owe anyone an explanation. We often provide additional or even unwanted information voluntarily. Aside from taking years off our own clock, we are also wasting the other person's time. That doesn't seem like a very nice thing to do. In fact, it's downright cruel at times, forcing someone else to sit politely and listen to you ramble. I haven't yet thought of an elegant way to tell someone to get to the point but if you have some ideas please share them!

And this goes for family too, you don't need to bare your soul just because you're related (unless you want to). Yes, there is the consideration of honesty with your partner (at times) but if you're an adult your mother doesn't require an explanation even if she demands one.

19   James Altucher. "The 20 Habits of Eventual Millionaires." *Medium*, Mission.org, October 12, 2015. Accessed February 9, 2021 at https://medium.com/the-mission/the-20-habits-of-eventual-millionaires-9329f95ec78d

91

Collage

This simple distraction is both fun and provides a good excuse to hoard magazines. Collect all the images that turn your crank and put them in one place. There are a million or more ways to do this but most options use images, either electronic or in printed form. You can collect images of the actual things you want or just images that represent your hopes and dreams. You can even gather up yummy images for no reason other than they just jumped out and grabbed you.

Take your images and post them on a board (either a real board with some kind of adhesive or on your computer) and then put it away to forget about it. Or toss it in a recycling bin. Or hang it above your desk to remind you what you're striving for. I've tried all of these options and each has its own unique rewards.

If nothing else happens, at least you spent some time on a delightful distraction while your child tears up an image of a black Lexus from Vanity Fair.

92

Compare leads to despair

I'm an expert in this area. If anyone can hold themselves up to another's seemingly impossible standard and then fail miserably to measure up, it's me.

I hold a master's degree in comparing; I could totally clean up on Sesame Street®. It's a hard habit to break but in the end, there is little or nothing to be gained by comparing ourselves to others unless you consider despair a gain. We use our comparison skills to our own detriment whether we consider ourselves the winner or not.

No two people, places or events in this world are similar enough to be evenly compared. We are an apple to everyone else's orange. Yes, both are round, and they are indeed fruit, but the similarities end there. Neither is better than the other, they are what they are, and are perfectly fine at that.

Comparing ourselves to others will not make us better, only miserable.

If you feel that you don't measure up, look for the ways you are comparing yourself or aspects of your life to someone else. Just recognizing the act of comparing is the first step to derailing the downward spiral.

93

Change your mind

You are not the sum of your beliefs and convictions. Often, we feel compelled to maintain an image of ourselves that other people have become accustomed to. We live our lives as Tess the Treehugger or Alex the Artist. Then a new idea presents itself and we begin to change our mind and change our ways. But if we change our mind, we might confuse everyone else! We're not predictable and easy to label anymore. We've broken our own mold.

New information finds its way into our life, into our brain, into our hearts and we just don't see the sense in our old beliefs. It's ok. We are human, we are fallible. Every now and then a huge wave comes along and washes us of all the things we thought we believed in; it erases who we thought we were—we become a blank canvas. This happened to me when I had a child, the experience completely deleted who pre-baby Laurie was. It's challenging to start over, to stare at the emptiness and not have any idea where to begin.

I'm still living in the state of beginning a new life and I've got nothing to hold on to at times. It will be interesting to see how this unfolds even though at times it feels like I'm staring at an uncarved block of wood. I like the way it looks right now; I don't even want to get out my knife and start hacking away. There is no rush to become anything or anyone

94

Don't take advice

Sometimes, when you've been fighting the good fight for some time and you've read everything and tried everything, and nothing seems to do the trick, it's good to just stop listening to other people. Take a break from trying to fix things, especially yourself. Sit back (figuratively perhaps) and observe the scene with fresh eyes.

As the only one who is near and dear to what you're going through, the act of patience may present a solution to you that no book or guru ever could.

95

Know your values

If you're clear about the values that are most important to you, it's easy to make even the toughest decisions. I discovered this concept in the work of Thomas J. Leonard, the grandfather of personal coaching and author of the excellent book *The Portable Coach*.[20] The aim is to identify your five top values and use them as a guidepost to navigate life's endless choices.

Discovering your values is not one of those lame, team-building exercises you're forced to engage in at work.

There are online applications designed to guide you through a simple process, so you can rapidly narrow it down to your top five. All you need to do is search for "Personal Values Test". It's fun to do and I've found my list of values immensely helpful when I'm faced with making one of those epic, life-altering decisions.

Because our core values tend to remain the same throughout our lives this isn't something you need to review on a regular basis unless something doesn't feel like a good fit. Like changing your mind, you can change your values if you want to. I had done this exercise before my son was born and even though becoming a parent turned my life upside-down like a table at a bar fight, my values have not changed.

---

20   Thomas J. Leonard. *The Portable Coach: 28 Sure-Fire Strategies for Business and Personal Success.* (Simon & Schuster, 1999).

Here's a list of mine to help you see the value in values: (That was corny, but I couldn't help myself).

Flexibility. This is why I'm self-employed, this is why I write. The 9-5 routine feels like a slow death to me.

Influence. I feel a profound need to influence other people. Again, this really comes through in my writing, hence the book you're reading now. If something I say causes a person to act or think differently, then that is deeply rewarding to me.

Beauty. I need to be surrounded by beautiful things and to make beautiful things. You might not agree with what I think is beautiful, but I don't care.

Simplicity. Complexity makes my head hurt. I get anxious if I spend more than thirty-minutes at Costco. My work, my life, my schedule, and my home need to be as simple as possible.

Fun/Adventure. In my opinion, everything should be fun or at least funny. Including books about depression. I haven't quite decided if I prefer fun over adventure, but I can always bend the rules and have both, can't I?

96

Share something deep

The best way to do this, if you don't have anyone close that you can really open up to, is to share something with a stranger. They've got nothing on you. They won't tell anyone you know. You don't even have to use your real name. A guy I knew was going through a challenging time. He was walking home from work, decked out in a custom suit and Italian shoes, when he strolled past a homeless person asking for change. My friend bought the stranger dinner and they both sat down on the curb to eat. They began candidly chatting and had a real connection over take-out.

When the conversation was over, the homeless guy, who probably hadn't showered in a month, hugged my friend before he went on his way. It was a moving experience and probably would have turned out quite differently if he'd just tossed the guy some change and continued on his way home.

When you share something deep it's like purging from the inside. You'll feel lighter.

97

Smile

Especially if you're grumpy and want to punch me for even suggesting this. Even if it feels fake at first just pull the sides of your mouth up toward your ears. It's kind of like a stretch for the face and as I've already explained, stretching is good for you.

This simple action actually alters your mood. The same is true for frowning or acting surprised although I don't know why you'd want to do that. If you think it's not working, look at something that makes you happy and smile at the image. Or just go around like a nut smiling at everyone you see on the street. This is the advanced application—I recommend doing this once you have mastered the art of the natural smile. If you walk around looking like the joker then someone might call the police.

98

Solve a puzzle

A puzzle doesn't have to be a 1000-piece reproduction of the night sky. Why set yourself up for failure on your first go? Do one of those really easy Sudoku puzzles, a kid's puzzle or a word search. I love those. They are designed for success. Completing one makes me feel like a genius. Get together with a friend and each of you create a maze for the other to solve. This can be a fun activity to do with kids too. If you're a puzzle master, then pick something challenging instead. No one will judge you because they don't have to know about the end result, unless you post it as your status update

The point is to get your brain working on something different.

Don't answer

(Phone/e-mail/text/whatever)

I find this one challenging. The best way for me to avoid responding to electronic beeps, rings, and notices is to turn all my devices off. Or give them to my son to play with who will break them or turn on some strange setting that I don't even know how to undo.

There are a number of reasons you might want to try this. It provides something simple you can control even when it feels you are living in a Rube Goldberg machine. It's also nice to have an afternoon free of distractions and can help you avoid dealing with people you don't want to talk to in the first place. Letting the phone ring and taking a few deep breaths instead reminds my body that it doesn't need to jump every time the outside world tries to get my attention.

The phone rings because someone wants to talk to me or sell me something. I let it ring because I am not obligated to respond.

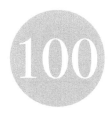

Play the love game

For this game it helps to have another person handy, particularly someone you like. Although, it could be transformational to do this with someone you despise, I think you should go easy on yourself.

The rules are simple. You and the other person take turns saying one thing you like/love about the other (depending on the status of your relationship). For long term feel-good affects, you can write down the qualities about yourself that the other person adores, just in case you're—I don't know— going through a rough time or something and a dose of cheer is required. This is a great game to play with someone you're close to but might not have really expressed how you feel.

If you're feeling shy you can play the game through e-mail or text messages.

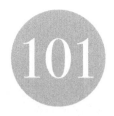

Plant seeds

Don't even bother planting them indoors unless you want to add to your disappointment. Let nature take care of your seeds! Besides, it's obvious that she's quite good at it, don't you think?

Do a little guerilla gardening and plant some native seeds in an outdoor area you frequently walk by. Something bright and cheerful would be nice - some wildflowers perhaps? If it's winter that's okay, plant them anyway. Nature is resilient. If you plant enough of them something will eventually grow. And if nothing grows you can just blame it on the weather instead of yourself.

Invest in earplugs

For a small fee you too can enjoy the peace and calm that simple, foam earplugs bring.

Now, they aren't going to cut out ALL the racket of a colicky infant but they "take the edge off", as my doctor assured me. Why I didn't think of them sooner is likely the result of mom-brain + sleep deprivation, but I am now grateful for the way they soften the ear-piercing effects of parenting.

Do not fear that you'll be unable to hear your child in distress, they merely turn down the volume of life so that you might hear yourself think. If you're the kind of person who is sensitive to noise this one tip could be a lifesaver. It works well for all parents by-the-way, not just moms! Everyone should have a foam ear plug collection tucked away in their bedside table, purse, gym bag or car. Heck just put earplugs everywhere. [Except where cats or children under three can reach them.]

103

Receive

There's a silly saying I'm sure you're familiar with:

It's better to give than receive.

This is total crap. First of all, in order to give, someone else has to receive. There's no way there can be more giving than receiving going on. I'm no math whiz but that seems pretty straightforward to me.

We need to receive in order to stay alive. Trees provide us with oxygen and shelter, the soil and plants provide us with food and I'm sure you get the point. Someone provides you with a paycheck or some kind of financial support but if you didn't receive it what would you live on? When you get a hug do you give one or receive one? Is it both? These are the profound questions of our time.

It's good to practice receiving because that's how you get the things you need and want. There are more than enough resources to go around, and when you refuse to receive you deny the giver the pleasure of giving. They will most likely just give to someone else instead.

Start by graciously receiving compliments or gifts with a simple, "thank you." No need to return the favor. I assure you there will be many opportunities for you to give of yourself today.

104

Little luxuries

A new lipstick, a cup of steaming tea, sitting by the water, reading a guilty pleasure, or listening to one for that matter. Money is not required to live in luxury. Luxury is treating yourself well; a deep breath among pine trees, a cold glass of water after a summer run, a hot bath with salts and lavender.

We have the opportunity to live in luxury every day even if only for a few moments. Find one way you can spoil yourself with a small indulgence today.

105

Hitting the wall

I don't know what you think hitting the wall means but I define it as an obstacle. A tall wall of thick stone blocking my path with no ladder in sight. When I'm starting something new, I tend to be blindly optimistic. Then I hit my first obstacle a few minutes later. Then I give up. Does this ring any bells for you?

I'm working on preventing it from happening to me by changing the way I look at obstacles. This idea is adapted from the work of a smart and successful guy named Dan Sullivan who coaches other successful entrepreneurs.[21] I often see obstacles as a sign that I should stop, I see it as a note from the universe that says:

"Dear Laurie,
Just wanted to let you know that this was
a really dumb idea and you have failed, yet
again. Way to go! When are you going to learn
you totally suck?"

Love,
The Universe

---

21   Dan Sullivan, "The Multiplier Mindset Blog." *Resources.* Accessed March 16, 2021, resources.strategiccoach.com/the-multiplier-mindset-blog.

So, here's what an obstacle really is— a thought that comes up in your mind. Yep, that's it, nothing but your opaque thoughts standing in your way. The thick, foggy glasses you've got on are making obstacles appear much larger than they are. Obstacles are a place where you have the opportunity to be creative and uncover an elegant solution. Obstacles are a sign that you need to grow a little in order to handle the challenges of the goal you're working toward. Embrace them because if you're doing anything worthwhile, they will show up with aggravating frequency.

106

Befriend other species

Trees, cat, squirrels, hedgehogs or, if you're brave—a Canada goose perhaps? They do not judge (except for geese, they are a**holes), and they don't care if you sometimes eat ice cream in bed or feed your kid organic vegetables.

Trees are great because they are (almost) always there for you. A column of reliability that you can count on. Somewhere safe you can return to and not as fleeting as summer birds. You can sit under one and read your phone while your child eats handfuls of mud and the tree won't give you a dirty look.

107

Do it your way

Are you overwhelmed by the insane magnitude of tips and advice for parenting from books and websites to family and friends? It's absurd the way we've turned parenting into a competitive sport or "the most important job you'll ever have".

It used to be that if your child lived to the ripe old age of 21, you were a monumental success. Somehow the bar has been raised so high that truly no one can conquer it. There will always be parents who think they've mastered the art of child-rearing but there isn't a human being among us who couldn't use some therapy so I would say they're delusional.

Take a break from looking outside yourself, step back from trying to "do it right" and do what feels right for you and your little one(s). You have inner wisdom to draw upon, a knowing that you can access if you're willing to trust it.

Sometimes the hardest part isn't figuring out what you need to do; it's dealing with the judgements and criticisms of others. But unless you're doing something unlawful or dangerous you need only reply with:

"Thanks for the advice."

(But I'm going to do it my way).

108

Just exist

There is no need to berate yourself for taking up air, water or space. I give you permission to just exist as you are. In the grand scheme of the universe we are tiny flecks in the cosmos. Our problems, our victories, the impact of our actions and decisions may seem monumental but they are—in the expanse of time and space—insignificant.

You don't need to be spiritual to appreciate how tiny even our seemingly massive planet is within the known universe. Imagine how small each of us appears in the eyes of the Milky Way.

For the next few moments you can just be, and that is enough.

The end

A friend suggested I wrap up the book in a powerful way. Maybe an inspiring story or a really great piece of advice. I think her idea is brilliant. Unfortunately, I haven't come up with anything yet but here is a quote I like:

"Life is a tragedy when seen in close-up, but a comedy in long-shot."[22]

— Charlie Chaplin

Free reader bonus

As a thank you for making it all the way through this book (whether you've actually read it or not), I've created free bonus material, including a video for you.

Please visit **https://www.ppdbook.com/reader-bonus** to access your goodies.

---

22   Charlie Chaplin. "Life Is a Tragedy When Seen in Closeup, But a Comedy in Longshot." *Quote Investigator*, October 2019. Accessed February 9, 2021 at https://quoteinvestigator.com/2017/02/05/comedy/.

Before you go

The trip to hell and back again after the birth of my son taught me a lot about compassion and vulnerability. I've done my best to share with you some of the tips and strategies I've scraped together so that postpartum depression might be less awful for other parents too.

I hope it helped you feel a little bit better, and a little bit less alone.

If you found even a small bit of joy in this book, would you mind taking two minutes to tell others about your experience with a review?

Any form of positive feedback means the world to most writers and also to those who look at the reviews before they decide to purchase a book.

A few positive words and a favorable star rating would make a huge difference to me... and to the many struggling parents we can reach together.

All the very best,

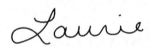

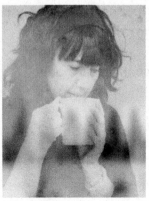

Author photo ©Laurie Varga

Laurie Varga is a writer, designer, mother, and mental health advocate. She lives in Canada and really likes soft, fluffy animals and drinking tea.

Find out more at **ppdbook.com**